Praise for - "Cerebral Eruption in Paradise"

"Illuminating! The reader joins [Merkel] in her day-to-day struggles and recovery." - (Daphne Dubois, New Hampshire Medical)

***

"Francine Feavel Merkel's, 'Cerebral Eruption in Paradise', recounts her personal experiences - providing answers to the many questions that brain trauma patients have." - (Ann Frommer, RN, MA, Columbia Medical)

Knowledge gained - "Cerebral Eruption in Paradise"

Before you embark on this journey, please know, the content of "Cerebral Eruption in Paradise" not only follows the life of Francine Feavel Merkel, but delves into the technical jargon as it applies to her aneurysm, multiple bone fractures, and recovery.

***

Whether you are a medical provider or an interested reader, it provides enough detail to describe the "how and why" of her maladies. Otherwise, disregard the medical-speak and walk in Fran's shoes through her 15 years of struggle.

CEREBRAL ERUPTION IN PARADISE

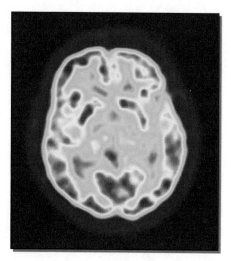

Scan Illustrates Power Utilization

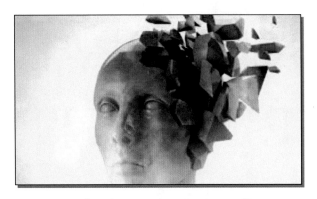

Cerebral Eruption in Paradise

A BRAIN ANEURYSM

RECOVERY

THE DARK SIDE OF MEDICINE

Francine Feavel Merkel

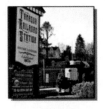

Vicann Press

Published by:

***

Vicann Press

9310 W. Riverside Ave.

Tolleson, AZ 85353

contact@frangives.com

***

First published by Vicann Press on August 8, 2016.

ISBN: 979-8-218-29734-3

ISBN: 90000

Printed in the United States of America

Dedicated to:

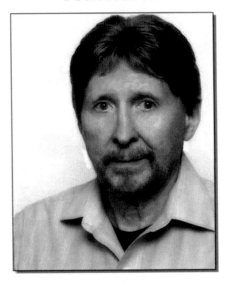

Victor Merkel

Husband, Friend, Lover.

Dedicated to:

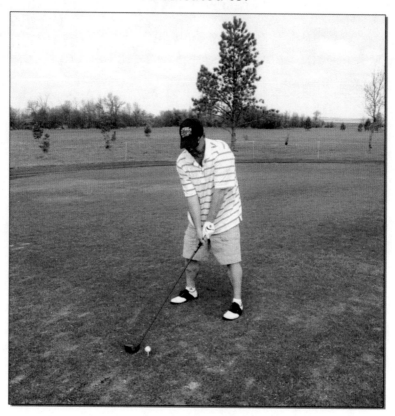

Ernie Feavel, Jr.

Ernie Feavel, Jr., brother, for love and support, above and beyond the act of human kindness.

He interrupted his life numerous times and traveled hundreds of miles to help me through the darkness. Ernie's influence guaranteed I received care from the best doctors.

He provided structure to my daily life, so I kept a positive attitude, ate the right foods, and worked hard to recover from my illness.

Introduction

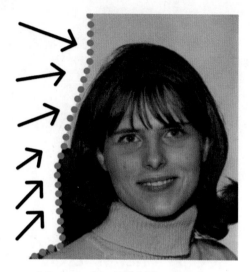

Memories Of Wisconsin

Since 1998, I tried to interest my husband, Victor, (then age 56) in retiring near Phoenix, AZ.

He chafed at the idea since his business had reached its peak in a booming economy.

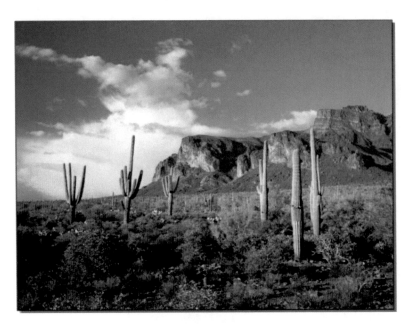

Arizona

When Victor reached 63, with reluctance, he agreed to help me manage the strenuous task of packing items we intended to keep and preparing for the sale of furniture, etc.

Also, planning the sale of his 19-year-old, sales & marketing business, required an even longer and more intense effort. Taking inventory, setting a price, and contacting potential buyers took months of preparation.

Special thanks to Tess Hill, Electronics Representatives Association and Attorney Gerald Newman.

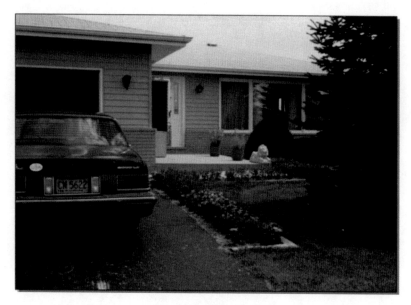

Genoa City, WI

Our Wisconsin home (4000 square feet), which we had lived in since 1979 (27 years), represented our heart and soul.

Every year, we improved some aspects of its construction, from adding air conditioning to siding, a new roof, a utility shed for our lawn tractor, dual pane windows and a swimming pool, etc.

After four garage sales, we sold all our furniture, lawn tractor, assorted tools, and equipment.

Exceptional gratitude to Don and Gail Holden, Brad and Ellen Bauman and others for their support.

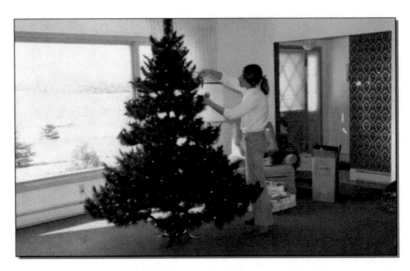

Christmas In Wisconsin

Finally, I sold most of my prized Christmas collection - angels, Santa statues and four Christmas trees.

In addition, we had to prepare our 7-year-old rental house for sale. The tenants had trashed the carpet with cigarette burns in addition to drilling holes through it to install sound equipment. Also, they broke a ceiling fan, pulled closet doors off their hinges, poked holes in the siding, trashed the air conditioner and damaged floor tiles in the bath/kitchen.

However, we had the last laugh when our rental sold for a tidy $27,000 profit. On the last day in Wisconsin, we celebrated wrapping up the last of our real estate sales.

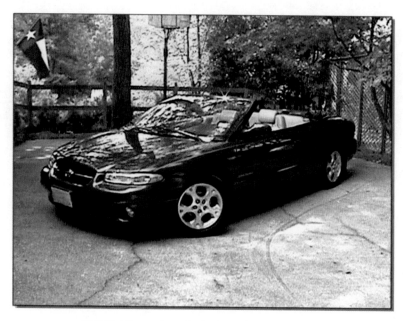

1997 Chrysler Sebring Convertible

We rented a car-hauling trailer for my second love, a 1997 Cherry Red, Chrysler convertible, and the remainder of our possessions.

However, when we started to load it, despite selling most of our furniture, etc., not everything fit.

With reluctance, we off-loaded the car and reloaded the trailer. This time everything fit. However, "Plan B" required me to drive the convertible from Wisconsin to Arizona.

Since I had a phobia about bridges, water and mountains, the trip ahead seemed overwhelming. In the end, I drove over 2000 miles, facing a combination of boredom on the mid-west's straight, flat roads to the sweats/racing heartbeat on the southwest's mountains and long span bridges. Thank God, no large bodies of water.

On the last days of our cross-country trek, my brother, Ernie, arrived at the house to install upgrades such as tile floors, marble counter tops, custom shelving, etc. Weeks earlier, we had planned for Ashley Co. to deliver new furniture, two days after our arrival.

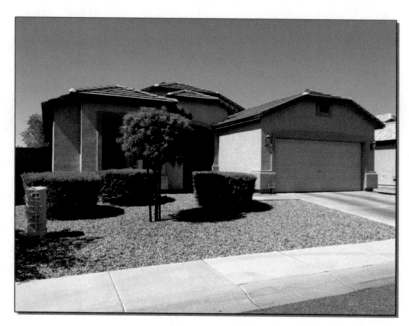

Phoenix, Arizona

When we pulled in at the new "Richmond America" house near Phoenix, AZ, our work shifted to motivating the contractor regarding repair of minor construction problems.

Next, we called on Shasta Pools for purchase and installation of an in-ground pool, work scheduled to start in several weeks.

Also, enlisted the services of a window blind company to measure and fabricate window blinds to be installed in about 6 weeks.

Finally, we joined a local gym (Litchfield - YMCA) to keep our schedule of exercise. Over the next month, we settled into a normal weightlifting and treadmill routine.

But fate had other plans for me. On the morning of March 26, 2006, I developed a raging headache on the left side of my head and shoulder. Everything went to hell from there.

Acknowledgements

Andy Feavel, brother, put his life on hold to provide moral support. As a 25-year National Guard veteran and Sous Chef at one of Wisconsin's top country clubs, he didn't hesitate to fly almost 2,000 miles to donate blood, provide encouraging words to keep my spirits up and run numerous errands both in the hospital and at home.

***

Arlynn Feavel Shaw, sister, provided warmth and caring as my BFF (best friends forever) and soulmate. Leaving her family, she cared for me through my darkest hours, provided chauffer services back and forth to the hospital, and bought numerous gifts to cheer me up. After my release from the hospital, Arlynn prepared all the meals and cleaned the house.

***

Paul J. Feavel, brother, interrupted his schedule to be at my side. As a cross-country, big-rig driver, he worked with his logistics scheduler to re-arrange his route. With his company's approval, he set a course to include Phoenix on his trip. While I lay unconscious in intensive care at the time, I'd like to believe my mind heard his familiar voice. Paul only stayed for a short period before the demands of staying on time caught up with him. Later in my recovery, when consciousness returned, I called him. Although I struggled to speak, he prayed with me.

***

Banner Estrella Hospital, built in 2005, serves the West Valley with medical services.

***

St. Joseph's Hospital, Phoenix, provides spinal diagnosis and surgery.

***

Banner Good Samaritan Hospital, Phoenix, provides lifesaving brain aneurysm surgery.

***

Airevac, provides emergency medical helicopter services for Banner Estrella patients.

Neurologist

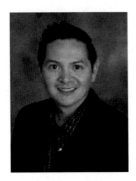

Dr. Troy Anderson

Dr Troy Anderson, neurologist, diagnosed post-surgery seizures and prescribed my anti-seizure medication.

In my opinion, he ranks at the top of his profession - excellent bedside manner, knowledgeable, and effective.

He attended Loma Linda University School of Medicine and completed his residency at the University of Alabama.

Neurosurgeon

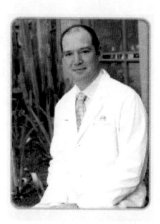

Dr. Byron Willis

Dr. Byron Willis, neurosurgeon, performed the critical task of repairing brain damage from my aneurysm.

He received his medical degree from State University of NY at Buffalo. Byron Willis, MD, completed neurosurgery residency at Cleveland Clinic.

He also holds chairmanship positions at Banner Good Samaritan hospital in Phoenix.

Contents

Chapter 1

FRONTAL ASSAULT ON MY BRAIN

SOMETHING IS WRONG, BUT WHAT

LOOKING FOR SPECIFIC SYMPTOMS

It struck me without warning at the Litchfield YMCA, as I did stomach crunches - a part of my daily regimen. A searing pain behind my left eye, plus trouble holding my head straight. It wanted to flop onto my shoulder and stay there. I also had an urge to throw up.

I looked for my husband, Victor, exercising in another part of the gym. I felt terrible yet still managed to communicate clearly about the pain. He drove me home and I climbed into bed.

A short rest provided no help and when Victor noticed my inability to string words together into coherent sentences, he expressed an urgency to get me to an emergency room.

Shuffling like an old servant, I ignored him and headed to the toilet. I sat there with no sense that I had critical brain trauma. In my injured mind, I felt annoyed with the altered perception of my world, but no more.

Only when my distraught husband pleaded with me to get in the car, did I reluctantly agree to join him for a trip to the hospital. At that point, I came to realize that something beyond my comprehension was wrong.

The following overview provides an unemotional and analytical comprehension of what to look for in the initial stages of someone having an aneurysm. An assessment will take a lot of the anxiety out of determining if a trip to the ER is warranted. However, even if just one symptom appears, you may want to err on the side of safety and see your personal physician as soon as possible.

Unruptured brain aneurysms, in most cases, stay undetected. These aneurysms, typically small, end up less than one half inch in diameter.

However, large unruptured aneurysms can, on occasion, press against the brain or its branching nerves and may result in various neurological symptoms.

I experienced headaches several weeks before my aneurysm ruptured, but in no way associated them with any critical medical condition. My parents, siblings and other family members never had an aneurysm.

Soon after my hospitalization at Banner Good Samaritan for the burst aneurysm, my brother, Ernie, underwent a brain scan, arranged by his personal care physician. His MRI did not find any symptoms of brain artery weakness.

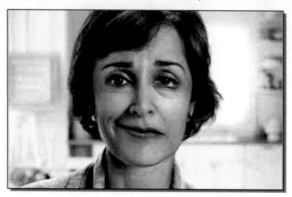

Aneurysm symptom, right or left facial muscles droop.

If you feel one or more of the following symptoms, regardless of age, seek immediate evaluation by a physician.

- Localized Headache

- Dilated pupils

- Blurred or double vision

- Pain above and behind the eye

- Weakness and numbness

- Difficulty speaking

My ruptured brain aneurysm resulted in a hemorrhage, which is defined as bleeding into the subarachnoid space. When blood escaped into the space around my brain, it caused sudden symptoms.

- Severe headache, the worst of my life

- Nausea/Vomiting
- Sudden pain behind my left eye

Although these were my warning signs after the rupture, if you are experiencing any of the additional symptoms listed: "Seek Emergency Medical Attention Immediately".

- Loss of consciousness
- Stiff Neck
- Sudden blurred or double vision
- Sudden change in mental status/awareness
- Sudden trouble walking or dizziness
- Sudden weakness and numbness
- Sensitivity to light (photophobia)
- Seizure
- Drooping eyelid

Chapter 2

PANICKED RUSH TO THE ER

GRAPPLING WITH BUREAUCRACY

DIAGNOSIS

REVIEW OF ANEURYSM TYPES

Before we reached the emergency room, my symptoms turned worse. Fortunately, my husband had thought ahead to bring a small plastic garbage can. It came in handy since I threw up several times and the pain behind my eye grew unbearable.

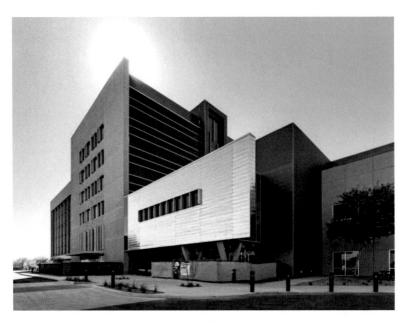
Banner Estrella Hospital

Since we had moved to the West Valley of Phoenix only a month earlier, Victor put his instincts and short-term memory to use. He sped down city streets toward a hospital we had seen from the 101 expressway a few weeks earlier - Banner Estrella.

Since it was early Monday morning, worker traffic clogged the streets but when we arrived, the ER parking lot sat almost empty.

Victor's vehicle screamed to a stop in front of the emergency room doors. He spotted a wheelchair near the entrance and brought it to my side of the Dodge. I struggled to climb on board and then, in a frenzy, he hot-footed to check-in.

I covered my left eye, trying to reduce the pain, while Victor grappled with the complacency of the hospital receptionist.

The woman kept looking at me to answer her questions about personal information - name, address, medical insurance, etc., even though it grew obvious to everyone, I wallowed in massive pain.

After confronting the nurse about the depth of my trauma, Victor took control of the communication, filled out some forms and pushed to have a doctor look at me immediately.

A nurse wheeled me, my husband in tow, to an ER cubicle, long enough to have a barrage of medical and insurance people ask Victor more questions. By now, I entered a world where my surroundings and their concerns evaporated. With calm indifference, I watched a steady procession of minions arrive to perform a CT scan, install a Saline bag, etc.

Later, I came to understand the serious nature of my doctor's diagnosis -- a brain aneurysm. Although ruptured aneurysms are relatively uncommon, they represent a very serious illness which is associated with a high rate of mortality and disability.

Looking back, having survived a ruptured aneurysm, I can say it was a very difficult experience to have gone through.

Even after ten years, I struggle to understand the medical aspects which led to March 26, 2006. Who is the culprit - genetics, unhealthy habits, etc.?

On an emotional level, sometimes I grieve for the beautiful life taken from me. In the darkness of night, I wake up in a cold sweat, alone and crying. Later, I thank God and Dr. Willis (neurosurgeon) for this alternate life, an exalted, life, given to me.

Now you know my experiences, on the first day of my aneurysm. Below, I've included an analytical review of aneurysms:

Gathering information about your condition can help ease this fear, begin the healing process, and bring a sense of comfort and support during a trying time.

An intracranial cerebral or brain aneurysm is a weak bulging spot on the wall of the brain artery, very much like a thin balloon or weak spot on an inner tube.

Over time, the blood flow within my artery pounded against a thinned portion of the wall. My aneurysm formed silently from wear and tear on the artery. As my artery wall became gradually thinner from the swelling, blood flow caused the weakened wall to bulge outward.

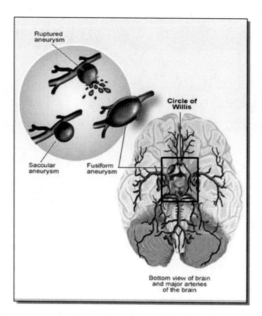

Ruptured Aneurysm, Circle of Willis

This pressure caused my aneurysm to rupture and allowed blood to escape into the space around my brain. It required advanced surgical treatment.

I experienced a saccular aneurysm, which is spherical in shape and involves only a portion of the vessel wall. They are frequently plugged, either fractionally or completely, by a blood clot, which is the most common type of aneurysm and accounts for 80% to 90% of all intracranial aneurysms. They are also the most frequent cause of non-traumatic subarachnoid hemorrhage.

A subarachnoid hemorrhage is bleeding into the space around the brain (the subarachnoid space). This occurs when an aneurysm ruptures. Subarachnoid hemorrhage from a ruptured cerebral aneurysm can lead to brain damage, stroke, or loss of life.

It is also known as a "berry" aneurysm, named for its appearance. It resembles a pouch forming at the "Y" division of veins with a stalk and neck. These tiny, berry-resembling bulges, take place at main "Y" and "branches" of the large arteries, at the brain's foundation, identified as Circle of Willis. "Circle of Willis" is a circle of vessels around the base of the brain where most aneurysms are found.

The fusiform aneurysm is an irregular shaped widening of a cerebral vessel that does not have a discrete neck or pouch on the wall of a liner. Fusiform aneurysms may burst, push on brain composition, or trigger strokes.

It is a rare type of aneurysm. It gives the impression of being like a pocket in a main wall on both sides of the artery or like a blood vessel that is expanded in every way possible. There is no stem associated with a fusiform aneurysm and it hardly ever ruptures.

Chapter 3

DOCTOR INFORMED ME – "ANEURYSM"

BLOOD VESSEL - "RUPTURED"

BLOOD ON BRAIN

SHIP ME BY HELICOPTER TO BANNER GOOD SAMARITAN HOSPITAL

Annoyed by the waiting, my perception of this place drifted off as I mellowed to a dimension with no boundaries. Lacking any edges, my mind bounced about without purpose.

In the meantime, Victor called my brother, Ernie, who lived about 40 miles north in Dewey, near Prescott Valley, AZ. He dropped everything at his work and drove to Banner Estrella Hospital.

After waiting for over an hour, the ER doctor came in and informed us that the X-rays revealed an aneurysm on the left side of my brain.

Since Banner Estrella had no neuro-surgery facilities for treating brain trauma, the attending ER doctor instructed his nurse to insert an assisted breathing tube into my airway and injected a coma inducing drug.

Inside my brain, I screamed, "Why are you doing this to me? Stop! I don't want something jammed down my throat." I sensed medical personnel hovering over me, forcing my mouth open and the sting of what must have been a hypodermic needle into my arm. I have no memory of the next 2 weeks.

Later, I learned that the nurse also packed me in ice and prepped me for Tweety Bird Yellow, helicopter transfer to Banner Good Samaritan Hospital on 12th Street in downtown Phoenix.

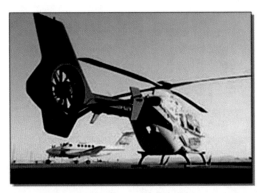

Tweety Bird Yellow, Medical Helicopter

An in-depth review of medical air transportation services:

Interest in some details of the helicopter ride would not enter my consciousness for many months later. However, at some point, I took the time to understand the inner workings of a paramedic air flight service. How do they mesh with hospital staff?

"Flight Medical Services" uses air transport to transfer patients. (FMS) personnel provide emergency and critical care to patients during evacuation. Helicopters are used to transport patients between hospitals and from trauma scenes.

Advantages of medical transport by helicopter include quick access to trauma centers. Helicopter-based, emergency medical service (EMS), also provides critical care capabilities during transport from hospitals to trauma centers.

An air ambulance is a specially outfitted aircraft that transports the injured in a medical emergency. These and related operations are called aeromedical.

Like ground ambulances, "air ambulances" are equipped with medical equipment vital to monitoring and treating the injured. Common equipment for air ambulances consists of computerized machines for assisted breathing, heart monitor, cardiac arrest resuscitation, gurneys, and medicine.

Chapter 4

BANNER GOOD SAMARITAN - PROCESSING

FELL OFF A GURNEY - ALMOST

I CAME HERE TO RETIRE, NOT DIE

ANEURYSM SURGERY

INDUCED COMA FOR 2 WEEKS

My husband informed me, weeks later, by the time he and Ernie arrived, I had been processed into BGS Emergency Ward. Over the weeks and months that followed, he reflected on events, good and bad, which occurred during my stay.

In his opinion, most of the staff members were professional and proficient. However, several incidents can only be labeled as inattentive, dysfunctional, or non-caring.

During the on-going preliminary testing and consultation with ranking medical staff, I almost fell off the examination table. Victor bounded to my side and held me while a lower ranking attendant centered me on the gurney.

Of course, I can't give a first-hand account of my craniotomy, but I'll try to give my take on the procedure. I received general anesthesia, so I never felt any significant discomfort.

The craniotomy was preceded by an MRI (magnetic resonance imaging) scan which provided an image of my brain which the surgeon used to plan the precise location for bone removal and the appropriate angle of access to the aneurysm.

The bone flap was restored to its original location using wire sutures.

Now that I've had my say, the following is a more detailed professional overview of my medical procedure.

Surgical procedure for clipping:

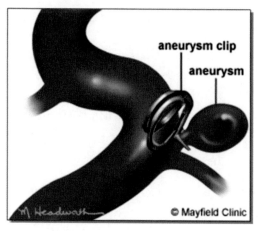

Courtesy Mayfield Clinic

Clipping Procedure

Clipping" is carried out by a neurosurgeon who will make an incision in the skin over the head, make an opening in the bone and dissect through the spaces of the brain to place a clip across the aneurysm where it arises from the blood vessel.

I was given general anesthesia, a breathing tube, then my scalp, skull, and the coverings of the brain were opened.

Since my aneurysm broke open (ruptured), it was an emergency that needed immediate medical treatment. My neurosurgeon's only option was surgery to clip the aneurysm.

Risks during the operation include breathing problems, reactions to medications, blood clot or bleeding in the brain, brain swelling, infection in the brain or parts around the brain, such as the skull or scalp, seizures, stroke.

Surgery on any area of the brain may cause difficulty with talking, recall, balance, sight, dexterity, etc. After-effects are sometimes slight or critical. Results can also be brief or permanent.

Signs of brain and nervous system (neurological) problems include behavior changes, confusion, loss of balance or coordination, numbness, problems noticing things around you, speech problems, vision problems (from blindness to problems with side vision), weakness.

After the Procedure: The hospital stay after aneurysm clipping is usually 4 to 6 days. But when bleeding, (my rupture) occurred before surgery, the hospital stay increased to over 2 weeks.

After successful surgery for a bleeding aneurysm, it is uncommon for it to bleed again. The long-term outlook depends on any brain damage which occurred from bleeding before surgery.

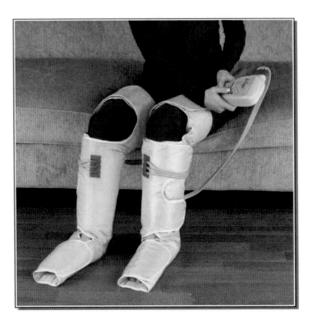

Anti-clot Leggings

Post-surgery, from the moment I entered "Intensive Care", the nurses installed pulsating leggings, to retard the creation of blood clots.

Also, "Radiology" inserted filters in my primary blood vessels.

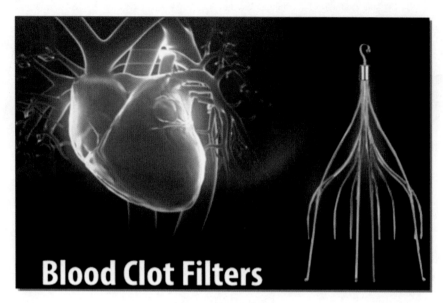

Blood Clot Filters

Anti-clot Filter

I think everyone has a general idea of the positive effects of clotting. However, the following (source Wikipedia) will give the non-medical person a smattering of technical background.

***

Coagulation is the process by which blood changes from a liquid to a gel. In most cases, it stops blood loss from an injured vein, then initiating a mend.

The mechanism of coagulation involves adhesion of platelets along with deposition of fibrin (protein).

Coagulation begins almost instantly after an injury to the blood vessel. Platelets immediately form a plug at the site of injury. Additional clotting creates fibrin fibers, thus reinforcing the platelet block.

Given the review of positive clotting, now look at the dark side of coagulation. For anyone who recently had surgery, prevention of blood clots is critical. Inspect your arms and legs for swelling, redness, soreness, or warm spots. Get to an emergency room if you have chest pains, fainting spells, or labored breathing.

Chapter 5

INCOMPETENT MEDICAL PERSONNEL

FIGHT TO GET PERCOCET

FAMILY AND FRIENDS REACT

My husband felt like a lost child amid those nurses running back and forth in the halls and in and out of rooms. In my opinion, they had no professional mandate to educate and inform patients and families of methods, procedures, and medications.

Needed medicine might not be given out, unknown to the patients or families. However, if a medication provided pain relief, you had to almost beg to receive it.

Also, diseases which were created from exposure to the hospital environment, ended up being po-pooed by doctors and stated as "normal" for this or that setting. This assurance didn't stop my family from languishing in their own fears about my developing thrush, blood clots, swelling, etc.

When a nurse could be flagged down and confronted about this, I was treated like a child whose hand had to be held. They said, "Don't worry about the blood clots."

Victor, in his opinion, couldn't stand for this type of shoddy treatment and reported it to the managing nurse. She listened patiently to this situation, but little changed.

The most gut-wrenching time of day for Victor came at 5:00pm, when nurses changed shift. He had to find my night nurse and beg her to give me Percocet. This is a pain killer which allowed me to get at least some hours of sleep.

***

I've listed some examples of incompetence, who assumes responsibility and your recourse to receive satisfaction.

If you are injured or abused when receiving treatment in a hospital, can you sue the hospital for negligence or medical malpractice?

• Hospital workers such as EMS, healthcare professionals can be sued for incompetent care. However, these personnel are not accountable, given a doctor's negligence.

• Normally, these workers are members of hospital staff. If the worker was performing job related activity, and harmed the health care client, the facility can be taken to court.

• On the other hand, if a doctor makes an error and hurts a patient, the health care institution assumes no liability for the health care professional's fault unless he is employed by the hospital.

In addition, if a facility staff member performs misconduct even though they are under a practitioner's direction, the doctor can be charged, without liability to the institution. Whether a member of staff is managed while the error transpired is determined by:

• If the practitioner was in attendance.

• Did the doctor have jurisdiction to stop the staff member's carelessness?

• A practitioner as a facility worker relies on the makeup of their association with the institution. Even though some doctors are facility workers, most practitioners are independent. As independent contractors, the hospital assumes no liability for their negligence, even if the misconduct occurred at the institution.

A health care provider is probably a facility worker, (not a contractor), if:

• The institution manages the doctor's employment time and holiday period - OR

• The facility establishes the rates the medical worker charges.

***

Exemptions: Once institutions are accountable for contractor practitioner's deeds.

- Under most circumstances, hospitals are not held accountable for an independent contractor practitioner's misconduct, except in undeniable conditions.

- When the facility does not present obvious information to a medical consumer that the doctor is a contractor, the patient can take legal action against the institution regarding the practitioner's unprofessional conduct. Hospitals steer clear of this predicament by notifying patients in entry documents that the doctor is independent.

Circumstances are not the same for medical clients harmed in the ER. Typically, the institution has no occasion to let ER patients know that a practitioner is a contractor. This liability allows emergency room patients to bring legal action against the facility because of the practitioner's negligence.

Several territories maintain the hospital accountable if employee rights are given to an unsafe doctor, regardless of their independent contractor status. The institution is also accountable if a competent practitioner, for whatever reason, turns inept.

Chapter 6

NURSES ROUGH OR UNINVOLVED

STRESS WITH FAMILY AND FRIENDS

GETTING OTHERS TO UNDERSTAND ME

ALWAYS MORE TESTS

My husband remained skeptical of the nurse's motivations. His opinion - they wanted to collect a paycheck more than fulfill their job duties as defined by Banner Good Samaritan hospital. Namely, care for the patients' wellbeing.

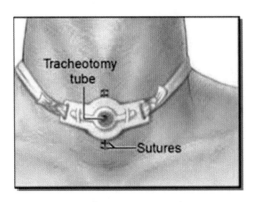

Tracheotomy tube

When I had a tracheotomy (a hole cut into my neck and oxygen tube inserted), the insertion point required constant maintenance. Bodily fluid accumulated at the mating surface and had to be wiped away, plus the sterile pad surrounding it must be replaced daily.

My husband was not allowed to change the pad but could wipe down the area with a cotton swab drenched in hydrogen peroxide. On one day, the accumulation was so bad, Victor asked the nurse to change the pad while she was there.

With no emotion, she said, "I have other patients, so it will have to wait."

Victor said, "Give me a fresh pad and I'll change it."

She said, "No, you can't change it."

End of discussion.

Here's an observation of nurses' burn-out:

It can happen to anyone. One day you like work, feel challenged by it and then a change creeps in. You have trouble focusing on work.

You may find your mind floating away to distant places when you should be focusing on your charting. You ponder important issues or insignificant musings. What do you want for dinner? Did I pay the phone bill? When is the perfect time to vacation in Hawaii?

Also, your mind-set has little to be desired. You used to have a helpful attitude. You wanted to improve the department. During burn-out, you grumble at any request.

You just want to do the least amount possible. You also welcome, with eagerness, any opportunity to go home early.

These changes can happen in slow measured steps, so you don't even realize it. You may be on the verge of burn-out.

Sometimes an exciting holiday is what you need to get a fresh start. A different environment can re-kindle the passion and cause you to focus on the challenge again.

Traveling, whether on a weekend junket or two-week cruise, may be just the change you need. Life is too short to complain your way through the day.

It seems that we are now seeing more and more examples of bad treatment and poor attitudes from hospital nurses.

It grows overwhelming, trying to stay positive and make allowances for the problems in health service.

When one keeps hearing negative examples of conduct. This problem seems even more bleak when listening to similar stories from patients just discharged back into the community.

Now back to my perspective:

There were so many distractions in a day, I'm exhausted just trying to keep track of them. The television would eventually rub me raw, mentally, with its constant drone. Nurses, nurses' aides, specialists, and the unending procession of ghouls drawing blood, taking x-rays and a multitude of other auxiliary tests.

With a constant rotation of medical personnel, they had to be re-educated to the nuances of my individual care. Not special care, but care in tune with my needs such as changing sterile bandages to insure of no infection. Also, to receive my pills on time without constantly reminding the staff.

Although the doctor performed amazing surgery, follow up on the many side issues were not discussed with the family. Victor had to complain to the head nurse about being brought up to date on my condition every day. In the end, the doctor held a meeting in my room, including all staff, to clear the air of any hard feelings.

Chapter 7

MOVE FROM INTENSIVE CARE TO REHAB

GRUELING SCHEDULE

WALKING, SPEAKING

While in the general population, it grew evident - the most irritating part of my journey, stood front and center. I had survived neurosurgery with successful results. The dire, alternative predictions of dying on the operating table or suffering major brain damage and ending up in a nursing home, did not happen.

My world went from passive, lying in bed all day to being periodically hauled out of my comfort zone to perform introductory rehab. When my short periods of rehab (15 minutes duration), about 4 times a day, met their requirements, the physical therapists approved me for full time rehab.

***

In my opinion, the transfer might have been a non-issue except for the dysfunction of communication between hospital management and rehab schedulers. The head hospital nurse on my floor scheduled me for transfer, not once, not twice, but three times. On the 3rd time, my husband wrote an internal complaint to the hospital manager in charge of patient logistics.

The manager hand-carried the complaint letter back to Victor along with a written letter of transfer. I was moved to rehab in the afternoon.

You have options, whether you're under 65 or over, to act on your treatment, if less than satisfactory. This includes conflict with doctors, nurses, counselors, therapists, financial people, to name a few.

During your hospital stay, the first contact for a complaint is your medical practitioner. Lay it out in detail and demand a response. Additional avenues of approach are facility social workers who assist in working out predicaments and finding help. Social workers put together assistance and documents at the time medical customers are discharged.

***

If troubled, finding correct care, document a grievance to the Joint Commission. JC confirms a lot of medical facilities' well-being and sanctuary training plus investigates patients' grievances. Joint Commission provides no medical supervision or billing.

***

Early release:

A source of anxiety for a lot of medical consumers is insurance coverage. They don't like extended waits. Get the attention of an institution release worker if you're not fully recovered. They will contact your practitioner.

Be aggressive, hire an attorney or independent medical billing watchdog to represent you. If the discrepancy is major, don't be pushed around and demand a fair and equitable resolution.

***

Therapy and Healing:

The relatives of those who lived through an aneurysm will possibly have hard choices and confronting events. Altered conduct, frame of mind and feelings are customary post-operation. A few medical clients, in addition, go through shortfalls in reasoning. Such changes present confrontations for medical custodians.

Caregivers are vital to effective treatment, so studying the concept of aneurysm outcome on conduct and body performance will assist your efficiency. Keep in mind, these transformations are brought about because of the aneurysm.

Healing a ruptured aneurysm requires tough and devoted encouragement from kin, plus rehab from practitioners and therapists. Getting the best treatment ensures improvement from brain damage.

***

Starting places:

Practitioners, nurses, or administrators offer the best resources to discover numerous treatment alternatives. Internet blogs and reinforcement teams dedicated to aneurysms prove helpful to medical clients who have endured an operation plus guardians assisting them.

Severe conditions happen when an aneurysm suddenly bursts and dictates an urgent operation. The bodily and mental results from unprepared, urgent surgery are solemn since the aneurysm has ripped open and injured the brain. Modest to critical restrictions are possible. Studies show exhaustion and frailness continue for a short time.

Also, stability difficulties, arm/leg frailty, problematic speaking, plus eye-sight troubles. Later, recovery from shortfalls improves in fragments or completely. It could take months or years to restore notable health.

Rehabilitation is essential to get back agility, verbal communication, and reasoning. Comprehending counselors, creating progress and incentives are vital.

A counselor identifies and takes care of medical clients with health difficulties and physical situations which reduce movement and performance. Therapists augment progress, advance healing and strength criteria which head toward fit and robust living.

Chapter 8

REGAINING PHYSICAL AND MENTAL STRENGTH

FIGHTING FEAR OF THE UNKNOWN

GETTING PEOPLE TO BELIEVE IN ME

GAINING RESPECT FOR MY EARLY WEAKNESSES

Each day, Victor and I packed up the car and pushed east on Interstate 10 headed for downtown Phoenix. We avoided the reckless drivers who changed lanes at high speeds, by staying in the HOV lane (2 people minimum).

Once we arrived, the hunt for a parking space near the rehab center started. Since I had a hard time walking, the long treks from the remote areas of the parking lot fatigued me.

Once inside, we had to wait ten to fifteen minutes in the lobby for our instructor. Most of the time, rehab professionals rotated so we never worked out with the same therapist twice.

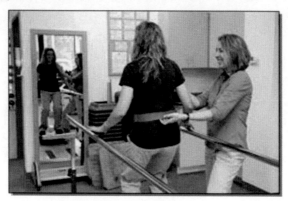

Rehabilitation

In the beginning, I performed a lot of walking, obstacle-walking (stones), stepping over barriers, ascending stairs, distance-walking, etc. They also ran me through occupational rehab which consisted of hand/arm and eye coordination. Putting together small puzzles, cooking food, etc.

Movements that most people took for granted were also part of the program - getting in/out of bed, sitting/ejecting from a couch, controlled falling and getting up. During a visit to the local zoo, instead of using a wheelchair, my brother rented a tandem bike, with him doing most of the pedaling. I contributed to the balancing.

Then on to speech therapy, which aggravated me when I struggled to make sense of words, spelling, numbers, and word games. These were repeated over and over for weeks, until I gained a sense of confidence.

This bothered me the most. I had been a mid-level manager at Motorola, responsible for supervising hundreds of people. I wielded authority in a fair and balanced way. The position required analytical skills, ability to interpret production numbers and communicate clearly.

***

An unemotional look at recovery:

Healing, (post-surgical follow up of an intracranial aneurysm) remains dependent upon assorted responses, regarding bleeding and the manner of ongoing attention.

Regarding a subarachnoid hemorrhage, the length of attention and recuperation are set according to severity of the damage, regardless of care. Post-subarachnoid hemorrhage - many medical clients will stay institutionalized for less than a month during which time they will be watched for progressive recovery.

Typically, up to two weeks after an aneurysm bursts, the veins near the bottom of the mind might develop tremors or contract. In critical cases, the outcome is stroke, and other problems such as accumulation of brain fluid. Excess liquid developing inside gaps of the brain, happens post - "aneurysm bursting" - and might endanger the patient's life.

Urgent action calls for positioning a hose to draw off the liquid. When the patient acquires difficulties or shortfalls because of the hemorrhage - therapy in or out of a clinic might be required. In favorable situations, numerous medical clients carry on prior interests in several weeks, lacking any restrictions.

Craniotomy entails a medical process of exposing the brain to clip an aneurysm. About 30 days are required to recuperate from this critical surgical procedure. Afterward, the medical client is mobile, however, refrains from forceful motion.

Medical clients tend their own nurturing and exercise to a degree of independence, ramping up pace, domestic activities, low bodily effort, etc. Following about 30 days, medical clients receive support to continue earlier actions. Stepping up movement helps patients continue their intensity and stamina.

A bumped-up danger always exists with a re-visit of the aneurysm. Following endovascular treatment, regular looking-after is needed. Medical clients go back for an angiography at random times for screening.

After an aneurysm with clip ligation, no scheduled looking-after is required, if elimination is documented.

***

Therapy and Recuperation:

The survivor's relatives manage hard choices and grapple with overwhelming situations. Deviation of conduct, disposition and feelings are universal post-operation. A few medical clients go through shortcomings in reasoning skills.

Variations offer altercations for nurses, etc., attempting to assist the medical client. The caretaker is important for recovery, so studying aneurysms and performance, plus bodily behavior, will help.

Keep in mind, variations are a product of aneurysm. The treatment of the medical client needs powerful and caring maintenance from kin, plus rehab from practitioners and counselors.

***

Access to data:

Your medical contacts are spokespersons for treatment alternatives. Internet and encouragement congregations, committed to support, are helpful. Maybe the prime starting place is with other surviving medical clients and successful counselors.

Chapter 9

UNDERSTANDING THE MOTIVES OF THERAPISTS

FINDING CHALLENGING ACTIVITIES

WHAT ABOUT THE REST OF MY LIFE

GOING HOME

I went through a learning curve trying to understand the motivations of nasty therapists. Only later did I come to understand their brutal regimen was a form of tough love. Their pushing me to higher levels meant regaining as much of my life as possible.

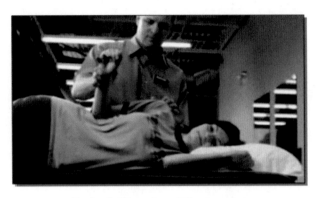

Rehabilitation Therapist

Over the course of several weeks, I started to know my rehab mentors, like old friends. Why they became therapists, their families, personal likes, and dislikes, etc. Above all, they considered rehab a profession, a calling to help people, not just a job.

As I reached a certain level of proficiency, my therapists found harder exercises to perform. Walks across a level floor were now passé. I trekked out to the clinic's front lawn and walked across the rocky terrain.

Also, I wore a web belt around my waist so the rehab person could grab it, to catch me before I might fall.

Learning to balance on unstable surfaces consumed a great deal of time on my final phase of rehab. They also used a computer-controlled platform that stressed my ability to maintain balance from the moment I stepped on it.

The following information reviews the many physical and mental maladies surrounding the aftermath of experiencing brain trauma.

***

Foreword:

Your brain aneurysm and therapy remain most important experiences, which persist post-release. The possibility of mental and bodily adjustments can be slight or major.

Recuperation, for medical clients with subarachnoid hemorrhage, has a propensity to be extended and complex, as opposed to non-rupture. The elderly and those with recurring medical problems recuperate at a sluggish rate.

Several of the post-aneurysm population need crucial treatment. Other medical clients grow independent, after a brief recuperation. Every circumstance is exceptional, and improvement differs.

***

Possible Shortfalls: Those who live through brain aneurysms could experience, brief or extensive, shortfalls. Given any situation, discrepancies recede at some point. Recuperation might take up to two years to overcome the shortfalls encountered.

Medical clients are advised to look for assessments from a specialist. They can establish the degree of performance and related difficulties. Concerning numerous situations, medical clients make use of communication, bodily and job therapists, to assist in recovery.

***

Detailed Discrepancies:

nervous system variations, eyesight difficulties, deficiency with odors, flavors, convulsions

***

Ordinary Difficulties:

incision aches and insensitivity, hearing loss, mouth tenderness, snapping sound in the skull

***

Broad Bodily Troubles:

head pain, change to "non-prescription" drugs, soreness, low energy, posterior tenderness, physically bound up, recall

***

Feelings:

sadness, bad temper, sidetracked, Identity, solitude, post-aneurysm despair

***

Therapy tips:

plan attainable objectives, look for a psychologist, work out a strategy with incentives, employment

Chapter 10

BACK HOME

CHECKED MY DRIVING SKILLS

SWOLLEN LEGS - TRIP TO ER

UNDERSTANDING SEIZURES

So many feelings jumbled up inside my brain as Victor pulled the Chrysler convertible into our garage. Home, home at last. I helped Victor bring clothes and assorted personal items, accumulated during my stay at Banner Good Samaritan hospital and the rehab center.

As I walked from the garage to our great room, I cried tears of joy. Nature saw fit to strike me down, but I survived and now I will rebuild the life that Victor and I intended. I swiped at tears and busied myself with chores, as woman of the house.

Next day, I decided to venture onto the road and test my driving skills. Although my husband felt reluctant to gamble with the family car, I sensed my mind and body stood ready to assume those duties.

I backed my convertible out of the driveway, put the transmission selector in drive and pressed on the gas pedal. It seemed to take forever; I didn't want to fail in front of my husband who looked on in gentle approval.

Later, Victor volunteered his Dodge, 4 door sedan, which he had used while a sales executive at Vine Sales, Inc., near Chicago. However, I think he followed his heart, confident the car was in good hands.

My medical problems did not end when I returned home. Within twenty-four hours, Victor took me to the ER for swollen legs. They used a scanner to check them for blood clots. However, except for a lot of excess fluid, they checked out OK. A wasted but safety-first trip.

Soon after settling into a normal lifestyle, I grew comfortable with our new house and the warm Arizona weather.

However, unknown to me, seizures hidden inside my injured mind, lay in wait, ready to wreak havoc on my body. For the reader, if anyone you know had recent brain trauma, be aware of the following post-aneurysm conditions which are well documented.

Convulsions show up in a small percentage of medical clients experiencing mind trauma. Many attacks come to light within days after damage. Antiepileptic drugs are approved for a short time. They might lower the chances of a seizure.

For medical clients that suffer from a blood vessel rupturing within the skull -- the norm, from aneurysm to convulsion was 42 hours and the mean seizure was 2.4 minutes. Recurring spasms can follow.

Preventive medicine must treat significant mind trauma within days ensuing the damage, while an attack is greatest.

Medical clients, amid fewer premature fits may have less convulsions in the extended period. Furthermore, if early-on spasms happen, a sustained period of care is detrimental.

***

Assumptions: Unfavorable results from anticonvulsants are weighed in contrast to advantages in stopping distressing spasms. Now, proof leans toward brief, "elevated strength" drugs. Recommending anticonvulsants during the (excessive danger) phase, post-trauma, is an ordinary procedure.

Here's my take on the above medical-speak: Sometimes a rush to administer anticonvulsant treatment slows down the body's natural healing process.

***

EVERY PATIENT IS DIFFERENT AND PUTS THE BURDEN SQUARELY ON THE DOCTOR TO DO NO HARM.

Chapter 11

SURPRISE! RUDELY INTERRUPTED BY SEIZURES

FINDING A NEUROLOGIST - FAST

THANK GOD FOR TRILEPTAL

EXPERIMENTING WITH VALIUM, ACUPUNCTURE, ESSENTIAL OILS

GETTING PUMPED UP AT THE GYM

I grew accustomed to a routine in the comfort of my home. Getting up on my own, dressing, making the bed, breakfast, housework. Almost all the things I used to do, except climbing a ladder, running, lifting heavy boxes, etc.

However, finding a neurologist grew into my priority since I never had any warning when the first seizure overwhelmed me. Victor panicked, screaming at the 911 people, and arriving EMTs.

My life swung full circle in less than 30 days, except my trip to Banner Estrella now included an expensive ambulance ride.

Everything is different but, in some ways, the same. Nurses and doctors poking their heads into my ER cubicle. My husband, whose demeanor always entailed a calm brooding, now paced the room like a caged animal.

My second seizure, witnessed by the attending nurse and my husband, came without warning. I was told that Victor reached toward me as if to put his fingers in my mouth. One of the nurses grabbed his arm and saved him from getting his fingers bit off.

Fortunately, Dr. Willis recommended a neurologist, Dr. Anderson, who has training in managing disorders of the brain.

Dr. Anderson gave me immediate care for seizures by prescribing an anti-seizure medicine - Trileptal. He also prescribed a companion drug - Cyclobenzaprine, which acts as a muscle relaxant. In a consulting role, he treated my ailment and then advised Dr Hoang (primary care) of my neurological health.

Since the quality of my life depends on the daily use of these drugs, I have reviewed them here for your evaluation.

TRILEPTAL

From Wikipedia

Trileptal is an anti-epileptic drug available as 150 mg, 300 mg, and 600 mg film-coated tablets for oral administration. Oxcarbazepine, (marketed as Trileptal by Novartis), is a white to faintly orange crystalline powder.

***

Possible side effects of oxcarbazepine (Trileptal):

hives, difficulty breathing, swelling of your face, lips, tongue, or throat.

Oxcarbazepine (Trileptal) can also reduce the (sodium) in your body to dangerously low levels, which can cause a life-threatening electrolyte imbalance.

***

Contact your doctor right away if you have:

headache, trouble concentrating, memory problems, weakness, loss of appetite,   feeling unsteady, confusion, hallucinations, fainting, shallow breathing, severe seizures.

CYCLOBENZAPRINE

From Wikipedia

Cyclobenzaprine, brand name ("Flexeril") among others, is a "muscle relaxer" medication used to relieve skeletal muscle spasms and associated pain in acute musculoskeletal (system, enables movement) conditions. It is the best-studied drug for this application.

***

Medical Use:

Cyclobenzaprine is FDA-approved to treat such muscle spasms associated with acute, painful musculoskeletal conditions.

It decreases pain in the first two weeks, peaking in the first few days, but has no proven benefit after two weeks.

ACUPUNCTURE

One of the alternative treatments I've tried is "acupuncture". During my search for relief of pain, I overcame my previous bias with non-medical procedures and kept an open mind. The therapist I chose held numerous degrees and taught acupuncture at a local college.

For me, the results with several weeks of treatment seemed hard to quantify. I felt positive, because at least I tried to improve my condition. However, looking back, the pain in my back and legs seemed unchanged.

I told the therapist and she decided to try something more advanced. This required the acupuncture needles to be inserted in certain points on my upper torso. Within a short time, I felt dizzy and weak in the legs.

My brother and husband kept me from falling and contemplated calling an ambulance. Since Victor had experienced a few of my ER visits with "no" conclusive result, he opted to wait and see if it subsided. After fifteen minutes, all my symptoms disappeared. I never went back.

However, I can't ignore the documentation supporting the effectiveness of acupuncture, in some limited areas. You will find below an unbiased summary of this complementary practice to western medicine.

Acupuncture

From Wikipedia

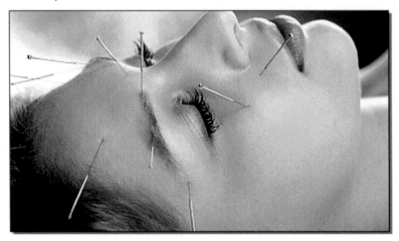

Facial Acupuncture

Acupuncture (from Latin, acus (needle) and punctura (to puncture) is a form of alternative medicine and a key component of "Traditional Chinese Medicine" (TCM) involving thin needles inserted into the body at acupuncture points. It can be associated with the application of heat, pressure, or laser light to these same points.

The method used in TCM is likely the most widely adopted in the US. It is rarely used alone but rather as an adjunct to other forms of treatment. TCM theory and practice are not based upon scientific knowledge, and acupuncture has been described as a type of pseudoscience (practice presented as scientific but fails to meet norms).

The conclusions of many trials and numerous systematic reviews of acupuncture are largely inconsistent. An overview of Cochrane reviews (independent organization, classify medical research info) found that acupuncture is "not" effective for a wide range of conditions, and they suggest it may be effective for "only" (chemotherapy-induced nausea/vomiting), (postoperative nausea/vomiting), and (idiopathic headache - increased pressure within the skull).

The most common mechanism of stimulation of acupuncture points employs penetration of the skin by thin metal needles, which are manipulated manually, or the needle may be further stimulated by electrical stimulation (electroacupuncture).

Needles vary in length between (0.51 to 5.12 inch), with shorter needles used near the face and eyes, and longer needles in areas with thicker tissues.

Apart from the usual solid acupuncture needle, other needle types include three-edged needles and hollow hypodermic type needles. Japanese acupuncturists use extremely thin needles that are used superficially, sometimes without penetrating the skin, and surrounded by a guide tube. Korean acupuncture uses copper needles and has a greater focus on the hand.

ESSENTIAL OIL

"Essential Oil Therapy" had always seemed a bit questionable to me. But I agreed to keep an open mind.

However, on a trip to explore specialty stores, red flags popped up in my mind. The attendant asked me to perform some spiritual movements of my arms. According to the young Asian girl, their gyrations indicate which oil will perform best. My first and last visit.

The only scent I tolerate is an occasional spray of Lilac room deodorizer.

That said, I well understand the existence of a powerful industry which produces and distributes numerous "essential oil" products.

Also, users are in the millions, worldwide. They believe these oils produce some "positive" effect. For the curious among us, I've included an overview of the process and specific oils.

***

Essential oil

From Wikipedia

An essential oil is a concentrated liquid containing volatile aroma compounds from plants.

Oil is "essential" in the sense that it contains the essence of the plant's fragrance - the characteristic fragrance of the plant from which it is derived.

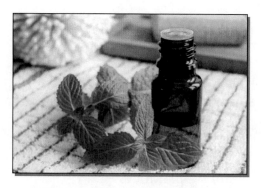

Peppermint Essential Oil

Essential oils are also known as volatile oils (capable of being transported to the olfactory system in the upper part of the nose), ethereal oils (synonym for volatile oils, evaporate readily from aromatic plants), aethereal, (steam distilled from plant material, soluble in ethanol, fermented sugar/alcohol) or simply as - oil of the plant from which they were extracted, such as oil of clove.

The term essential used here does not mean "indispensable" as with the terms (essential amino acid) or (essential fatty acid) which are so called since they are nutritionally required by a given living organism.

Essential oils are generally extracted by (distillation) of separate substances by evaporation-condensation, often by using steam. Other fragrance extraction processes include:

• "Expression" - extraction specific to citrus

• "Solvent extraction" - use of solvents, (petro, ether, methanol, etc.), to extract odoriferous (fat loving) lipophilic

• "Absolute oil extraction" - solvent extraction, highly aromatic, oily mixtures

- "Resin tapping" - incising (cutting) pine trees to collect sap
- "Cold pressing" - plant is crushed, the resulting paste is pressed to separate liquid oil from solid material

They are used in perfumes, cosmetics, soaps, and other products, for flavoring food and drink, and for adding scents to household cleaning products.

Oils are volatilized (diluted) in a carrier oil and used in massage, diffused in the air by a nebulizer, heated over a candle flame, or burned as incense.

PAIN RELIEF

Prescription Medication

While searching for relief from constant pain, my doctor prescribed a small dosage of Valium (medication produces a calming effect). I enjoyed some relief, but the drug left me groggy.

After complaining about my feeling sleepy all the time, he suggested Lyrica (treats neuropathic pain) Although it provided some relief, the drug left me with an off feeling. I discontinued it a few weeks later.

***

Neuropathic pain

The "European Federation of Neurological Societies" recommends pregabalin (Lyrica) as a first line agent for the treatment of pain associated with central neuropathic pain (dysfunction in peripheral nervous system).

Other first line agents, including gabapentin (neuropathic nerve treatment) and tricyclic (antidepressant chemical compounds) antidepressants, are given equal weight as first line agents, and unlike pregabalin, are available as less expensive generics.

EXERCISE AT THE GYM

Since I had been a devout follower of body-building exercise at a gym, in the end, all paths led back to working-out my upper and lower muscles. However, my previous experiences had been as a trauma-free person, not someone with a deficit, trying to get back to normal.

Medical clients must take it easy starting physical actions and maintain reduced force when working out. However, never curtail training. Exercise to repair the wound, plus avoid potential damage. Stay aimed at higher aspirations.

Progression will vary over time - extra movement and diverse muscle training. Changes will be made to focus on the areas needing improvement. Limbering up and recuperation are most significant.

No matter that the damage is from a brain aneurysm, working out hastens improvement. Keeping fit the whole time speaks to quick recovery from any vulnerability.

Recuperation and restoration: exercises extending the limbs, lots of sleep, hot/cold body washes are mandatory to healing.

Nourishment hurries curing. Muscle mass requires nourishment with meat, vegetables, etc. The wounded physique needs a steady ingestion of protein.

Vitamin and mineral intake: To restore muscle mass, reinforce initial healing tenderness and create collagen (protein in tissue), a regimen of the following must be consumed - iron, copper, magnesium, calcium, zinc, manganese, and major vitamins.

Getting adequate slumber - the physique's top protection is sleep. It takes part in a significant function - renewal after damage. The physique produces significant hormones crucial to a robust resistant organism, increased muscle mass and bone potency.

Harboring a lousy outlook - viewpoint is a substantial part of the recovery process. The medical client must display an eagerness to get healthy. Get ready to work with the trainer and give 100%.

Chapter 12

YEAR 1

ATTITUDES, PREJUDICES, LIKES, DISLIKES

PHYSICAL NIMBLENESS, EYESIGHT, DENTAL

MULTITASKING

With 12 months behind me and experimenting with all the prescribed drugs and treatments available, I came to understand that only a select few had any beneficial effect on my day-to-day life.

All the others fell into my "Questionable List". Meds for blood pressure, blood thinner, pain, etc. And all of them had side effects, some of which caused vomiting, dizziness, sleepiness, a high feeling, distortion of my personality, swelling of my face or jaw, etc.

A combination of feelings ran through me, denial, anger and just not caring, but despite these negative emotions, I pushed forward, and my physical capability continued to improve.

STATE OF MIND

Mind trauma alters the medical client's feelings. Brain damaged survivors possess several disturbing troubles.

Problems managing sensations - medical clients encounter feelings rapidly, however, they are short-lived. The survivor also experiences (lability), a yo-yo effect - cheerful to depressed to enraged.

***

The reason? Frame of mind (moving back and forth in emotion) is often brought about with medical injury to the mind which manages actions.

Kin might seem puzzled - did they, somehow, insult the injured person? The mind brings about unexpected periods of giggling or weeping.

Disturbing flare-ups have no connection to their actual thinking. Like "chuckling" upon hearing a distressing story. Medical clients have no influence over their passions.

***

Medical clients must have a discussion with their psychologist to discover the reason and take care of their changed emotions. Guidance for kin permits them to deal with it also.

A few drugs alleviate this frame of mind. Seek advice from a practitioner who specializes in mind trauma. Kin must stay composed when flare-ups take place.

The medical client must go to a peaceful spot and seek composure. Accept their point of view and allow them to discuss their concerns. Offer advice when the medical client recovers. Change the topic of conversation to something lighter, when possible.

* * *

Apprehension - worry, perceived as larger than reality. Mind trauma survivors are frightened, lacking any sound reason. Mistakes, failures, and criticism top off the list.

Challenges to the new psyche - noisy crowds, being hurried, abrupt difference in activities. Several patients experience devastating spells.

Fear might be linked with a traumatic circumstance. For a while, the setting which brought about the trauma, gets repeated and disturbs slumber. Angst (worry) requires individual therapy from a psychologist.

Fretfulness after mind trauma - trouble interpreting their surroundings, baffles medical clients, causing difficulty in working out obstacles. Patients grow inundated with choices. Apprehension occurs with a lot of demands and little time.

* * *

Solution to nervousness - Decrease surrounding challenges, which might bring about worry. Support the patient with a relaxed demeanor, to lower their angst.

Daily, their schedule needs planned behavior - training, focused gatherings of like-minded patients, etc. Medications can help bring ease, also psychiatric help, or both.

Depression - a common reaction to major adjustments in their life. This way of behaving materializes throughout later recuperation phases, when sensitive to the circumstances.

Devastating thoughts - get in the way of improvement. Signs of despair - gloomy, lack of slumber, not focused, isolation, sluggishness, suicidal. Brain injury can cause depression within several months after the trauma, but not right after.

Sources of melancholy - when a medical client works to change, hopelessness can begin short-term or permanently depending on their previous status with kin or the public. Despair takes place when the wound is exaggerated in the mind of the patient. Depression can be caused by biochemical and physical changes. Common treatments for hopelessness are (drugs and/or psychoanalysis).

***

Yoga and aerobics - alleviate gloominess. Sadness doesn't represent limitations or responsibility, only sickness. Medical clients can't just walk it off - search out therapy near the beginning.

***

Anger - Kin depicts the medical client as having a quick trigger or going ballistic at the drop of a hat.

Over 70% of traumatic brain injury patients have bad tempers. They shout, curse, destroy property and commit violence.

The reason for this crisis - damage to sections of the mind which manage feelings. Aggravation and unhappiness concerning changes in existence, career loss and self-sufficiency. Lonely, miserable, unfocused, no recall and inability to articulate.

***

How to treat tantrums - dropping anxiety and lessening frustration eliminates anger. Mind trauma patients must study (rage-managing, self- soothing) leisure and improved exchange of ideas.

Refrain from submitting to their difficulties. Establish interaction guidelines to advise the patient - shouting, intimidation and violence will not be tolerated. Otherwise, cut off communication with the patient. Later, in a quiet moment, discuss what motivated the medical client to react. Advise positive responses as alternatives.

UTILIZING EXERCISE GEAR

Fitness centers offer an assortment of machines for resistance, cardio and/or free weights. Your exercise schedule can be varied, creating a successful overall program.

A fitness center supplies all the equipment for constant development, from novice to highly developed.

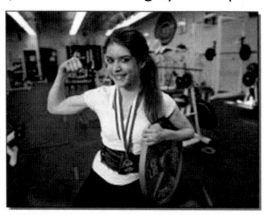

Fitness Center

Apparatus will vary among exercise rooms, but some standards are universal for acquiring helpful exercise.

***

Resistance Equipment

Peruse the placards. Fitness apparatus label the proper areas under attack. A widespread error is to replicate similar body group exercises in the same session. Case in point - if you use the leg press procedure, don't use the leg curl procedure.

Regulate the device appropriately. A lot of gear permits fine-tuning of the seat posterior or elevation. A few have cushioning, crossways and upper-most of the knees. Machines that engage junction flexion (bending of a joint) might have a rotating position to complement. Correct fine-tuning by a coach (at least the first time) is necessary to prevent harm.

Pick a load and pump no less than eight replications, but don't exceed 12. Try to complete no less than two sets on each apparatus and when 12 reiterations grow effortless, increase the burden, or attempt an alternative work out. Don't train on the identical contraption for more than two weeks, or six successive gatherings. Physique will grow familiar to the identical effort and will evade muscle growth.

Apply a measured movement while exercising on gear and experience the full breadth of movement unless informed differently. Manage your motion and keep tightness by ending while the load just about makes contact.

***

Cardio Equipment

Begin limbering up. No matter if you favor performing complete cardio exercises immediately, after a strength work out, or prefer to mix it up, limber-up for five minutes preceding any resistance instruction. Stationary bikes and treadmills perform well for a fast stretch since an increased heart rate isn't essential currently.

Climb on and start your progress. Excluding the treadmill, a good number of cardio machines want you to begin (peddling or stepping) prior to an indication to get started.

If you're just preparing on a fresh apparatus, use the physical adjustment for most of the period.

Launch the treadmill at the same time as you have your feet on the side runners. Begin at a gradual pace and grasp the handlebars as you initially begin moving. Raise the pace and angle as you improve.

At all times, keep a correct figure with posture erect and abdominals tight. Maintain shoulders at attention with head upright. Back neck, and pelvis must line up. Make use of handrails, however, never prop your body against them. Loosen-up and unwind for a few minutes afterwards. A lot of equipment will perform these methods routinely.

***

Free Weights

Exercise with barbells or dumbbells to drive triceps, biceps, and deltoids. Increase resistance to lunges and squats by means of dumbbells lowered at the sides or a barbell across the shoulders.

Choose weights that challenge your resistance and perform comparable repetitions. Challenge yourself by means of slanting and declining worktables for curls and presses.

CATARACTS - DIAGNOSIS AND TREATMENT

A condition that my optometrist had predicted years ago, started to appear. My eyesight had degraded to the point where I struggled to read everything. Smoking and the trauma of my aneurysm contributed to the clouding of my lenses. My cataracts had to be removed.

***

Cataracts

From Wikipedia

Cataracts are most commonly due to aging, but may also occur due to trauma, radiation exposure, birth defect, or occur following eye surgery for other problems. Risk factors include diabetes, smoking tobacco, prolonged exposure to sunlight, and alcohol. Either clumps of protein or yellow-brown pigment may be deposited in the lens reducing the transmission of light to the retina at the back of the eye.

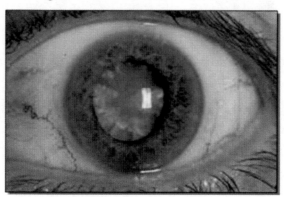

Cataract Patient

***

Cataract - a clouding of the lens in the eye leading to a decrease in vision. It can affect one or both eyes. Often it develops slowly. Symptoms may include faded colors, blurry vision, halos around light, trouble with bright lights, and trouble seeing at night.

This may result in trouble driving, reading, or recognizing faces. Poor vision may also result in an increased risk of falling and depression. Cataracts cause half of blindness and 33% of visual impairment worldwide.

***

Diagnosis by eye examination:

Prevention includes wearing sunglasses and not smoking. Early-on, the symptoms may be improved with eyeglasses. If this does not help, surgery to remove the cloudy lens and replace it with an artificial lens is the only effective treatment. Surgery is only needed if the cataracts are causing problems. Surgery generally results in an improved quality of life. Cataract surgery is not easily available in many countries, which is especially true for women.

About 20 million people are blind due to cataracts. It is the cause of about 5% of blindness in the United States and nearly 60% of blindness in parts of Africa and South America. Blindness from cataracts occurs in about 10 to 40 per 100,000 children in the developing world and 1 to 4 per 100,000 children in the developed world. Cataracts become more common with age. About half the people in the United States have had cataracts by the age of 80.

DENTAL CARE

From Wikipedia

I waited months before deciding to get a new dental exam from Dr. Clausen in Avondale, AZ. I had too many physical and emotional issues to sort through, resulting from my aneurysm. So, I kept pushing concerns about my teeth to the bottom of the list. I also neglected my dental hygiene with a hit or miss regimen. When I finally made my visit, Dr. Clausen discovered fresh cavities. Since they were small, he didn't have to inject a numbing agent and immediately took care of them.

Unfortunately, with involvement of the federal government in my dental coverage plan, I was later forced to change dentists.

***

Teeth maintenance

Teeth cleaning is part of oral hygiene and involves the removal of dental plaque (mass of bacteria) from teeth with the intention of preventing cavities, gingivitis (inflammation of gum tissue), and periodontal (plaque induced inflammatory condition) disease.

People routinely clean their own teeth by brushing and flossing using small brushes, plastic picks, and water flosser. Dental hygienists can remove hardened deposits (tartar) not removed by routine cleaning. Those with dentures and/or natural teeth may supplement their cleaning with a denture cleaner.

***

Brushing

Careful and frequent brushing with a toothbrush helps to prevent build-up of plaque bacteria on the teeth. Electric toothbrushes were developed, and initially recommended for people with strength or dexterity problems in their hands, but they have come into widespread general use.

The effectiveness of electric toothbrushes at reducing plaque formation and gingivitis is superior to that of conventional manual toothbrushes.

***

Flossing and interdental cleaning

Cleaning between teeth may help to prevent build-up of plaque on the teeth. This may be done with dental floss or interdental brushes. 80% of cavities occur in the grooves, or pits and fissures, of the chewing surfaces of the teeth. Special appliances or tools may be applied to supplement toothbrushing and interdental cleaning. These include special toothpicks, oral irrigators, and other devices.

***

Professional teeth cleaning

Teeth cleaning (also known as prophylaxis, literally a preventive treatment of a disease) is a procedure for the removal of tartar (mineralized plaque) that may develop even with careful brushing and flossing, especially in areas that are difficult to reach in routine tooth brushing. It is often done by a dental hygienist.

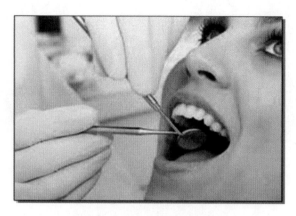

Professional Cleaning

Professional cleaning includes tooth scaling (removing dental plaque), tooth polishing and debridement (ultrasonic instruments, hand tools and chemicals), if too much tartar has accumulated. This involves the use of various instruments or devices to loosen and remove deposits from the teeth.

Most dental hygienists recommend having teeth professionally (cleaned) every "six" months. More frequent cleaning and examination may be necessary during treatment of dental and other oral disorders. Routine (examination) of the teeth is recommended at least every "year".

This may include yearly, select dental X-rays. They are used for "dental plaque" identification and removal. Good oral hygiene helps to prevent cavities, tartar build-up, and gum disease.

Chapter 13

YEAR 2, 3

BLOCK WATCH

HOMEOWNERS' ASSOCIATION

Entering the second year, I grew more comfortable with my life. And just like my previous service as "board supervisor" in Bloomfield Township, WI, I assumed a new government role as "block watch official" in Tolleson, AZ.

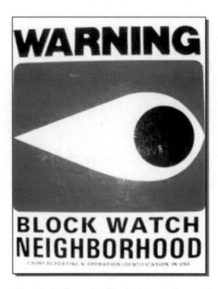

Block Watch Neighborhood

I hand-delivered "Block Watch" literature to every house within 4 blocks of our avenue. I gained the friendship and trust of most homeowners. However, some neighbors had no interest in the organization. Over time though, several of those homeowners turned to me when they had problems such as break-ins, defaced property, or complaints about ordinances, etc.

A great benefit of this position is buzz about news in the area. I found that our neighborhood grew saturated with drugs. If juvenile delinquents had enough energy, the hoodlums broke into homes and started fires, stole TVs, stereo equipment, appliances, copper pipe from air conditioners, etc.

The juvenile delinquents also excelled at vandalism; if they knew a house had been vacated through foreclosure, etc., the criminals threw stones, busting the windows. After the glass, they threw bricks and large stones at the walls, knocking out stucco, leaving divots in its place.

***

Definition of Block Watch - fellow citizens with an agenda and concern for the safety of neighbors. This includes collaboration with law enforcement to decrease misconduct plus make living better.

***

Homeowners' Associations - official unit formed to keep up shared regions. They can also impose title limits.

Nearly all new property growths have HOAs, typically produced once the expansion is constructed.

***

Covenants, Conditions & Restrictions (CC&R's) are given out to property holders. HOAs guarantee and uphold the superiority and worth of real estate assets.

Chapter 14

YEAR 4, 5

CATCH PNEUMONIA

FALL AND BREAK HIP

HOSPITAL AND SURGERY

REHAB AT SPOONER

PUMP UP AT GYM

As my recovery entered its fourth year, I felt a need to reach out to friends and neighbors in the area, offering help, if needed. Sometimes they just wanted a shoulder to cry on or advice about how to handle a problem.

One of my friends ended up in the hospital with a respiratory condition. Of course, I comforted the poor soul during my visits and brought food, soda plus dessert. The grateful patient preferred it to the typical hospital food.

Since hospitals provide breeding grounds for hostile bacteria, I tried to keep my hands washed and take reasonable care not to contact common surfaces. However, despite my best efforts, pneumonia filled my lungs and rendered my body defenses weak.

This insidious virus took its time, showing up as congestion on the first day and my temperature rose to 102 degrees by the second night. My husband planned to take me to the ER the next morning if the fever hadn't come back down.

I ended up at the ER about 3:00am, however my husband didn't take me. Waking up in the middle of the night and feeling listless, I struggled out of bed and headed to the kitchen. I made it to the refrigerator before losing my balance. I fell backward, hitting my elbow on a door hinge and fracturing my femur on impact with the tile floor.

Victor tried to lift me, but I was in too much pain. Determined to move me to the RAV4, he found a large baggage cart in the garage and managed to slide me onto it. We reached the open SUV door and since he works out at the gym, I expected him to lift me the short distance to the passenger seat.

However, the pain was so intense, he lowered me back onto the cart. I noticed his sad eyes as he pulled out a cell phone and dialed 911.

I ended up at Banner Estrella for the next several days while hovering in a twilight world. A pulmonologist forced oxygen, at a rate of 20 liters, into my lungs. He needed to implement procedures to counter pneumonia.

A nurse administered antibiotics and arranged for a chest x-ray. The results confirmed massive congestion in the lungs. Also, a technician dispensed Albuterol through a drug delivery system called Nebulizer to treat breathing.

A surgeon evaluated how to repair my fractured femur. The doctor took several MRIs to determine the type and location of titanium rods.

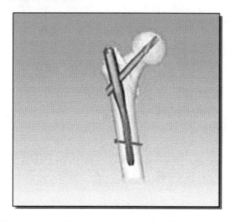

Femur, Titanium Rods & Screws

Last, a neurologist took x-rays of my brain to ensure the fall did not incur any damage.

I fell from a standing position, resulting in damage.

The femur fracture was "Transverse" (uninterrupted horizontal line going crossways. No misalignment or shift. No skin or muscle tears.

Symptoms:

Instant, acute hurting. Can't walk on the wounded leg, undersized and crooked.

***

Practitioner Assessment:

- Explain the nature of your incident. This data assists in deciding the extent of injury.

- Elaborate on your overall fitness and list medical problems plus prescriptions.

- Following a chat about damage and health, a practitioner performs an assessment of your overall condition plus damage.

Your Physician Examines:

- The apparent irregularity concerning your appendage abnormal slant, curling or reduction.

***

Additional Physical Diagnosis:

- The practitioner determines the length of your leg and thigh, gazing for irregularities - tautness of the membrane and tissues in the region of your thigh. They will also examine for abnormal heart beats. When alert, the physician checks for feeling and flexibility.

Examination Using Imaging:

- X-rays: A widespread method for assessing a break.

They give comprehensive visuals of the bone area. X-rays prove if bone remains whole or busted. Also, the kind of break and location in the femur.

- Computed tomography examination: If the practitioner wants additional information, they arrange a CT scan. It illustrates segments of the extremity, highlighting the seriousness of the break. Bone cracks might be fine and difficult to distinguish on x-ray as opposed to CT.

***

Therapy:

- Most femoral shaft fractures need an operation to repair the damage.

***

Medical Care:

- Point of surgical procedure. Given the tissue remains intact, the physician will delay the operation until the medical client is settled.

- In anticipation of your operation, the practitioner will immobilize the extremity. The damaged bones need to be lined up straight and length maintained.

- Traction consists of a winch structure of weights and counterweights. They keep the broken sections of bone as one. Traction also maintains your appendage in the right position and reduces soreness.

- Intramedullary nailing. Presently, the technique doctors utilize to take care of femoral shaft fractures is intramedullary nailing. During this process, a custom metal bar is placed in the marrow channel of the femur. The bar supports the fracture, maintaining the arrangement.

- An intramedullary nail is placed in the channel, hip/knee via a small cut and attached at mutual terminations. Nail and bone are kept in correct locations throughout mending.

- Titanium is used for Intramedullary nails. The nails are manufactured in assorted spans and widths to match femur bones. Intramedullary nailing offers tough, durable performance.

***

Recuperation:

- Nearly all femoral shaft fractures undergo up to six months to entirely mend.

Impact On Leg Stress:

- Numerous physicians promote leg activity near the beginning of recuperation. Stick to the practitioner's advice regarding stress on the hurt leg.

- On occasion, physicians let medical clients place heavy stress on the leg immediately. Inversely, the patient might be required not to stress the leg in anticipation of the fracture mending. Stick to the practitioner's directives cautiously.

- As the patient starts moving, they might need the aid of crutches or a walker.

Bodily Rehabilitation:

• The medical client will experience a drop of bodily power in the hurt region. Workouts are vital throughout the therapeutic procedure. Rehabilitation brings back vigor, movement, and suppleness.

• I performed all my rehab at Spooner Clinic across from Banner Estrella Hospital in Avondale, AZ.

Rehabilitation also concentrates on soreness release, encourage mending, and bringing back performance. During initial treatment, a counselor assesses the reason for tenderness and builds up a tailored arrangement.

• Increase motion

• Decrease tenderness

• Return performance

• Avoid additional harm

Counselors also use supplementary healing techniques, modified to the specific requirements of every medical client. They apply practical methods to employ manipulation to the affected areas. These include ultrasound, electrotherapy, Fire/Ice bags, etc. Furthermore, they teach medical clients to self-train.

***

Operation Setbacks:

• The procedure itself, blood deficiency, anesthesia difficulty

• Damage to nerves

- Sluggish curing fractures
- Peg friction against tissue and metal staples

Chapter 15

YEAR 6

FALL AND BREAK SHOULDER

DISASTER AT BANNER THUNDERBIRD

REHAB AT SPOONER

PUMP UP AT GYM

During the 6th year of my recovery, I felt like a battle-hardened soldier. I carried the scars of my aneurysm and fractured femur like WWII hero, "Audie Murphy", with pride and humility.

I thought the traumatic events of my life had come and passed. However, the old myth of bad things happening in groups of three loomed over my head like a dark fog.

With our lives settling into a normal routine, Victor and I decided to have the house painted. In Arizona, after 7 years, paint starts to fade and doesn't provide full protection from the elements.

We enlisted the services of my brother, Ernie Feavel, Jr., to spray paint the exterior of our house and hand brush the trim with 100% acrylic latex. He had to travel from North Dakota, so I prepared the spare bedroom for him.

On the day before he arrived, I scrambled to clean up the back yard, remove our dog's (Butch) poop and tidy up some loose items. While returning to the back door, I didn't raise my bum leg high enough and tripped on a raised edge of the patio.

I fell forward on the cement, hitting my head and shoulder. Victor called Daphne, my neighbor, someone who has been like a sister. She soothed me while Victor arranged for an ambulance.

At Banner Estrella, the ER doctor informed me - the impact fractured my left shoulder plus an X-ray of my brain, raised concern of bleeding. Last, my oxygen concentration ran in the high 80s. Normal is the high 90s.Later, they transferred me to Banner Thunderbird. Upon arrival, I discovered the night nurse, in my opinion, had the demeanor of an Army drill sergeant. Despite the pain, I instructed the grumpy, "bedpan cleaner" to back off.

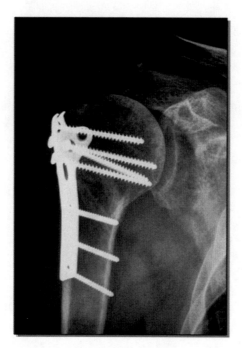

Shoulder, Titanium Plate & Screws

During my stay, Dr. Tony Nguyen, surgeon, repaired my shoulder with a titanium plate and screws.

In addition, the pulmonologist kept me on 20 liters of oxygen and slowly reduced it to three liters. Last, the neurologist monitored my brain for potential bleeding but found none.

***

A Medical Evaluation of Shoulder Construction:

Two other "shoulder bones", are connected by soft tissues (ligaments, tendons, muscles, and joint capsule) to form a raised area for the arm to work.

• The fall fractured (broke) the "proximal humerus" (top of the upper arm bone).

- The peak layer is the "deltoid muscle", (muscle just underneath the skin), which gives the shoulder a circular appearance.

- The "frame" of the shoulder is covered by several (stratums of soft tissues).

Specific Findings of My Proximal Humerus Fracture:

- Directly under the deltoid muscle is "sub-deltoid", (liquid -filled pouch), like a water balloon.

- A severely swollen shoulder.

- X-rays found a fractured top of the humerus.

- Very constrained movement of the shoulder.

***

Severe Pain:

Since the pieces were shifted out of position, a surgical procedure was required. My operation involved securing the splintered remains with a plate and screws.

***

Life After My Shoulder Injury:

My day-to-day routine was affected for several months. I required a period of immobilization followed by rehabilitation at Spooner.

"Spooner Physical Therapy" is a private outpatient rehabilitation practice dedicated to helping individuals restore function and movement.

Shoulder workouts were part of my managed physical therapy plan. Training increased flexibility, improved breadth of movement, and helped me recover muscle power.

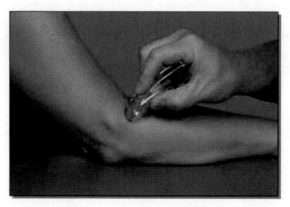

Assisted Soft Tissue Mobilization (ASTYM)

Also, my therapist (Carolina) started "ASTYM" (assisted soft tissue mobilization) using a special tool for assisted massage.

Developed by a team of professionals, this procedure yields long-term results with short-term therapy, even when other treatments have failed. Only ASTYM-certified therapists may carry out the ASTYM treatment.

Chapter 16

YEAR 7, 8

INSIGHT INTO MY LIFE

KEEP MOVING UP

FUNCTIONAL RECOVERY

Starting in year 7 and through 8, I kept pushing the limits of my physical and mental strength. Although I slow-dance with my husband on occasion, I have accepted the fact that I will never rock and roll with the powerful gyrations of my youth.

Victor pursued a full-time writing/publishing career in 2006, authoring 2 biographies, 1 young adult novel, and co-authoring 3 WWII historic novels with Ann Frommer, https://sites.google.com/site/annfrommerhome. He creates word pictures that inspire the imagination. During quiet moments, I can write clear and understandable sentences but can't make the words sing.

However, I have developed a talent for numbers and self-taught the basics of Quicken. I use it for all our financial tracking. I set up all our online bill-paying for the easiest and quickest method depending on the capability of the service provider.

I have been so busy with my own challenges, sometimes I neglect to watch the many patients stricken down with only one illness, in quiet submission, they drift off into the sunset. They become invisible, isolated, and alone. I feel the most helpless for these lost souls.

My sister-in-law recently passed away after struggling with a medical condition. Although she lived several thousand miles away, we talked on the telephone. I often wonder - if I had been there to help her, would she still be alive?

***

Value Of Family:

Providers are concerned regarding distress on relatives and end up researching appropriate help groups. Assistance agencies are available for kin, helping them to admire the relative's strong points while enduring difficulty. Counselors improve relative's initial consciousness using their assets to deal with shock and sustain constancy through it all.

Relatives "implies" multiple people, somehow connected, either racially, officially, hereditarily, or psychologically. Kin safeguard, sustain and nurture the individual to excel.

Bodily damage is scary and devastating to the relatives. These occurrences violate the communal gist of well-being. Each family goes through shock in a different way. However, it is connected to collective feedback.

Distress alters households while trying to endure their situation. A patient's pain crashes into their relatives' comfort zone and affects their interaction and performance.

Medical clients go through the consequences of a shocking incident. Versions extend from toughness to recurring physical conditions, head pain, slumber problems, stomach troubles, elevated blood pressure or psychological problems, acute nervous tension, PTSD, etc. In adults of all ages, these symptoms can slow developmental growth or change the course of one's life.

Mature sex can "intensify" calm handling of distressed incidents and consequences. However, when income, etc. are floundering and nervous tension is elevated, couples have trouble sharing feelings. In the extreme, this might lead to divorce.

Relationships with close relatives are essential to recuperation. Security and assistance will hurry improvement. However, if elder kin have their own health problems, they might not be supportive to their offspring, producing negative performance.

Brother and/or sister interactions are a significant basis of friendship, particularly if sharing the same tense surroundings. However, if the strain is too extreme, siblings grow burdened and competition spirals upward to a major fracas.

A comprehensive array of "personal connections" can give encouragement to get well. Kin estranged from family can build a different set of connections. Folks alienated for their own protection must generate hard decisions on future relations.

Relatives supply the means for basic requirements: well-being, provisions, refuge, and ongoing maintenance. Distressing conditions exhaust assets, (capital/vigor), reducing chances to gain knowledge and pursue a career.

Typical obligations are - expensive legal actions, transfer to smaller quarters, adjustment training. These cause a shortfall of revenue plus fewer occasions with relatives. Kin struggle to conduct schedules and support their way of life.

Emerging consciousness of the shock on kin, plus their responsibility to an offspring, emphasizes the family unit orientation.

Once kin perform customary habits, they escalate resilience. Chatting, smiling, remembering good times plus teaming up to get to the bottom of difficulties, handling tension and schedule activities.

When kin encounter multiple ordeals, a "beaten down" result requires "shock" examination plus implement therapy.

Chapter 17

YEAR 9, 10

LOOK FOR HAPPINESS IN EVERY MOMENT

I PLAN FOR NOW AND THE FUTURE

IF I'M IN PAIN, I WITHDRAW TO A COMFORTABLE PLACE

My psychologist trained me to reach a calm mind-set. I make peace with both sides of my brain and feel grateful for the enjoyment of food, drink, and good friends.

With a start to the new year (2016), I complete my tenth year of living, post-aneurysm. Although every day is an unknown venture, I vow to bulldoze through any pain, anxiety, or depression to the other side.

And what lies on the other side, you might ask? Well...an 8-hour period filled with productivity. This might be paying monthly bills, documenting info for our income taxes, up-keep of the house and yard, record-keeping of Victor's writing income and expenses from his business.

Of course, no life is perfect. During quiet periods, I try to reconcile my losses with the positives. Sometimes I win, other times I lose. I consider it a work in progress.

***

Regarding a critique on mind damage and its mending, a religious viewpoint must be added. This review offers experiences with the associated rehabilitation.

Also, steady cerebral babble might persist from well-meaning family and friends. As a result, the medical client feels rejected and inferior. By trial and error, they discover meditation to reduce frustration, which changes her outlook on life.

***

Training for relaxation: Non-conventional healing, post-cerebral damage, is achieving official status in institutions. They consist of acupuncture, reflection, biofeedback, massage of the sutures, etc.

The public incorrectly compares an injured mind to a hurt arm or leg. Trauma, yes, but also including the neurological aspect.

My personal challenges were remembering people's faces, names, places, and past events.

Combined therapy helps medical clients. This field is still being studied to better understand the process.

Conventional practitioners use combined therapy as a supplement to traditional treatments.

The cranium has a range of motion, the length of its sutures. If the rhythm is uniform, the mind remains fit. Therapists loosen these limitations to return the beat to routine.

Sometimes, I can't remember people, places, or activities. However, you can choose any type of internal reflection, mantra, calming pictures, etc., to retrieve those elusive memories. Control your breathing and feel liberated from the world around you.

***

Your makeover. Shortly after finding consistent internal reflection, medical clients profited. They shrugged off their confusion and felt in control of their environment.

Friends and family feel welcome again and the patient feels no need to retreat. With a strong motivation and tolerance for excitement, their viewpoint is positive.

When medical clients become educated on internal reflection, it assists them to be cognizant with feelings and contemplations.

Patients are aware of deep inhalation, soothing their psyche and gaining knowledge. They can dismiss ways of thinking and be upbeat. Internal reflection can be a substitute for medicinal rehabilitation. Many medical clients recuperate from despair. Worry drops off and vigor returns.

Further investigation revealed that internal reflection alters the mind by dropping steroid hormone concentrations, linked to anxiety. From my own experience, I have yet to confirm this.

***

Fresh links to your personality and friends, family. Investigation reveals mental "ability-based" treatment, also assists patients to bond. Loneliness declines considerably.

Treating head damage might create quality occasions with family. Therapy might also open someone up to find other talents, replacing their old vocation.

The influence of desire in healing. Harmony of the soul, body, and mind can create a powerful force. By means of conviction, one improves the course of action.

A lot of patients talk regarding religion. Trauma survivors can reflect on their existence as out of the ordinary. They wonder about their humanity. Silence helps internal reflection to speed up recuperation.

***

In my opinion, while in surgery, I believe God appeared through a bright light. He asked if I wanted to enter heaven. Thinking of the loss to my husband and family, I answered no.

My next recollection was being told about the successful surgery. Every day, I thank him for returning me to my loved ones.

Inhale, exhale. Internal reflection requires only the focus of mind while customary medication maintains its time-honored role.

***

Ninety Second "Inhalation and Exhalation". Employ internal reflection to grow peaceful in the current instant.

Step 1. Grow Attentive

•   Be seated with foot bottoms relaxed, shut off gaze, focus on internal feelings.

•   Analyze the encounter.

•   Examine the reflections.

•   Look for thoughts.

•   Examine tense or rigid atmosphere.

Step 2. Bring together

•   Center on inhaling and exhaling, sense the stomach stirring, expanding, and contracting. Monitor the movement "in-out", fastened to a current instant.

Step 3. Spread out

•   Take in air, increasing consciousness and body awareness. Experience your whole mass throb with each breath.

Chapter 18

ADDITIONAL OBSTACLES AND SUCCESSES

In the search for understanding of what happened to me, starting with my aneurysm in 2006 followed by a fractured femur in 2010 and broken shoulder in 2012, I have read numerous articles and medical books. In addition, I have talked to people living with similar maladies.

Although I have been seizure free for 10 years, the threat of it is always in my mind. I have come to terms with the fact - I will have to take the drug, Trileptal or an improved alternative, for the rest of my life.

Along with controlling the misfiring of my brain comes associated pain. The companion drug, Cyclobenzaprine, muscle relaxant, used to reduce pain linked to seizures, has possibly overstayed its usefulness.

Finally, the years I spent smoking have caught up with me. Like a ninja, quiet and potentially deadly - COPD has enlarged my lungs and reduced the capacity to intake enough air to function normally.

I tried most conventional smoke cessation plans over a thirty-year period. This includes:

- Acupuncture
- One-on-one hypnosis
- Group hypnosis
- Computer scheduled cessation plan
- Nicotine patches
- Oral medication

Some had no effect; others gave me short term smoking cessation of 3 to 6 months. My most notable success was 7 years. However, when my mother contracted cancer, I started again.

***

In the last 2 years, my pulmonary specialist has added the following inhalers: Symbicort, marketed by AstraZeneca (combo formula - treats asthma & COPD) and Advair, marketed by GlaxoSmithKline (combo formula - treats asthma & COPD).

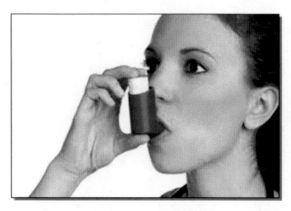

Symbicort Inhaler

Chronic Obstructive Pulmonary Disease:

(COPD) is a general illness of the lungs which causes difficult breathing.

*　*　*

There are two major types of COPD:

•   Chronic bronchitis, which includes mucus plus a continuing cough.

•   Emphysema, which has to do with harm to the lungs over an extended period. Most individuals amid COPD possess a blend of equal circumstances.

*　*　*

Causes:

•   Cigarette use is the major reason for COPD. With increased smoking, statistics indicate a person will develop COPD. However, a percentage of the population can smoke for a long time and never get COPD.

- In extraordinary circumstances, nonsmokers who are deficient in a protein called (alpha 1) antitrypsin can acquire emphysema.

***

Additional threat issues for COPD:

- Contact with toxic gases or vapors in the place of work.
- Contact with extreme quantities of cast-off smoke and contamination.
- Recurrent utilization, of food preparation combustion, lacking appropriate dissipation in air.

***

Symptoms may include any of the following:

- Cough, accompanied by or devoid of mucus
- Exhaustion
- Respiratory illness
- Shallow inhalation (dyspnea) - grows dysfunctional amid minor movement
- Problem breathing
- Winded

Since the warning signs grow gradually, a small percentage of the population might be unaware of their COPD.

Assessment:

•   The top examination for COPD is a lung performance analysis named spirometry. This requires breathing out vigorously into a little instrument which examines lung capability. The outcome can be verified immediately.

•   By means of a stethoscope, taking note of lung performance can provide supporting information. However, on occasion, the lung function seems routine, but the patient has COPD.

•   Imaging analysis of the lungs, for example: x-ray and CT scan, offers further examination. However, by process of x-ray, the lungs might seem typical, despite established COPD. The advanced clarity of a CT scan has a higher probability of confirming COPD.

•   At times, a blood analysis named "arterial blood gas" might be prepared to determine the quantities of oxygen and carbon dioxide within the blood.

***

Therapy:

•   No cure exists for COPD. However, numerous remedies will alleviate warning signs and prevent the illness from progressing.

•   Quit smoking NOW. This will delay lung impairment.

Drugs to take care of COPD include:

•   Inhalers (bronchodilators) to assist opening the pulmonary passages.

- (Breathed in) or (by mouth) steroids to lower lung irritation.

- "Anti-inflammatory" drugs to reduce swelling in the airways.

- Specific "extended time" antibiotics.

***

In acute situations or through flare-ups, the patient might be given:

- Steroids (orally) or in a vein (intravenously).

- Bronchodilators in a nebulizer.

- Oxygen treatment.

- Help from an apparatus which aids inhalation: a mask, BiPAP (bi-level positive airway pressure), or by way of an endotracheal tube (inserted through mouth/nose).

Your doctor might recommend antibiotics for the duration of flare-ups since an illness can bring about elevated COPD.

***

You might require oxygen therapy at home when a depleted amount of oxygen is established in your blood.

Pulmonary rehabilitation can't heal COPD. However, it will educate the patient to breathe uniquely, to help resume a normal lifestyle.

Existing In the midst of COPD:

Listed below, health activities to prevent further COPD dysfunction, save your lungs from harm, and promote excellent health.

***

Hike to develop vigor:

• Question the therapist about walking limitations.

• Gradually build up the distance.

• Pass up conversation if breathing grows labored.

• Form pursed lip exhaling to clear out the patient's lungs ahead of the subsequent inhalation.

***

Activities to improve life at home include:

• Stay away from cold air or hot conditions.

• Avoid cigarette smoke.

• Moderate use of a fireplace and purge obvious household irritants.

***

Consume wholesome cuisine: poultry, fish, lean meat, plus vegetables and fruits. For those who struggle to maintain their weight, consult with a dietitian concerning higher calorie foods.

One option is an "operation" as an aggressive treatment for COPD. No more than several medical clients profit because of surgery.

- Emphysema - cut off sections of the unhealthy lung, which assists remaining branches to improve function.

- Lung transplant - only for most severe cases.

***

Viewpoint:

- COPD = a (never-ending) disease. This malady will spiral downward unless you quit smoking.

- With acute COPD, you will struggle to breathe during activity. If the difficulty grows critical, it might necessitate recurring treatment at a clinic or hospital.

- Speak to the practitioner regarding breathing equipment and end-of-life attention if the illness advances.

***

Obstacles:

Additional troubles

- uneven heartbeat (arrhythmia)

- heart swelling / failure

- pneumonia

- pneumothorax (uncoupling of the lung from the chest wall)

- critical weight deficiency

- reduction of bone mass (osteoporosis)

- weakness (debilitation)

- greater anxiety

Also, on an as-needed basis, my specialist prescribed the use of oxygen. At first, I rented an oxygen tank, which seemed appropriate at the time. However, I found the business principle, some oxygen distributors practice, is "profit only" - from insurance compensation.

In my opinion, some are jackals, feeding off the needs of those that require oxygen on a steady basis. I had to sign more paperwork than when I bought my car.

They also use intimidating wordplay. When I bought my own Devilbiss oxygen generator and wanted to return their rental unit, the first words out of their mouth, belched sarcastic, "OOhhh...you're refusing treatment?"

I grated, "You can call it what you want, but I'm returning this equipment, now."

The overweight, snippy clerk flitted about, processing paperwork while ignoring me. She smacked the cancellation invoice on the counter in front of me along with a pen.

I took my time reading the form to make sure no under-handed clauses hid in the fine print. When satisfied, I signed and pushed it back to her. The clerk, red faced, ripped off the second page and threw it toward me. It was my copy of the "Return of Equipment" document. Done and done.

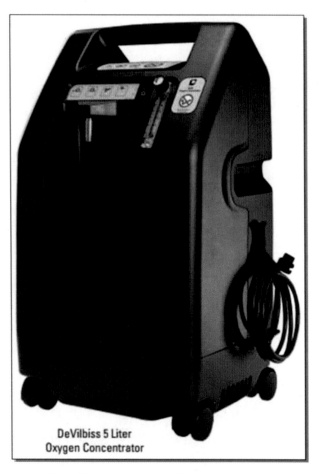

DeVilbiss 5 Liter
Oxygen Concentrator

Devilbiss Oxygen Concentrator

Satisfied with the form, I uttered a dull, "Goodbye.", and mentally washed my hands of the place. I also informed my pulmonologist about their unprofessional attitude.

In hindsight, I noticed the oxygen company also raised their monthly rental rate. If I had paid 6 months of increased rental payments, I would be out of the money and own no oxygen equipment. However, I DID buy a new Devilbiss unit direct from the manufacturer and those 6 rental payments, paid for it.

There are businesses who prey on medical clients, the patients who are trying to recover from a malady. You need to either be your own champion or have one available, to make sure doctors, nurses, medical suppliers, etc., treat you fairly.

* * *

I hope the technical information and my experiences written on these pages will illuminate your path. No matter what the motivation for reading "Cerebral Eruption in Paradise", either as a patient, relative, medical provider, therapist, etc., you can reach an understanding of the other's perspective. From that moment, you will move forward with courage, optimism, and confidence.

END

Biography

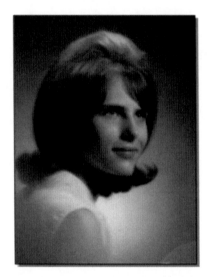

Appleton West High School

Appleton, WI

The beginning of my wonderful adult years started after graduation from AWHS. Victor and I met through family members, dated, married, and moved to the Chicago suburbs.

We rented a small apartment and started our new life.

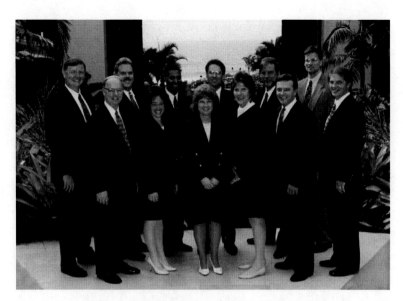

TCS Land Mobile Products Sector

Hawaii, Kauai Island

I joined a Fortune 500 communication equipment company, Motorola, and took advantage of their generous higher learning program -- "Motorola Education Center" and climbed the ranks of management.

My position allowed me to direct the efforts of numerous men and women engaged in the processing of communication equipment. My favorite perk involved business travel to major Motorola facilities across the US.

The final legacy, I leave behind, is helping them to create a start-up, Motorola/Rockford, IL, focused on expanding their North American capabilities.

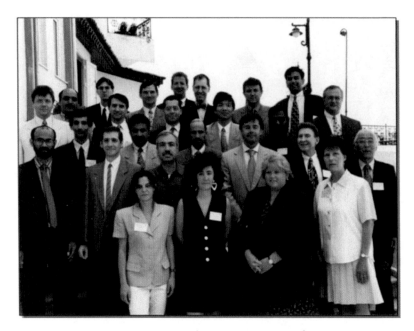

WTN International Business Conference

Kusadasi, Turkey

After 29 years, I changed careers and joined Victor in his sales and marketing company. As VP Sales, I used my organizational skills to help secure an agreement with an international sales and marketing franchise. We traveled West Europe and the Middle East (before 9/11), developing business contracts, to sell products in the US.

Our biggest partner manufactured and distributed industrial products in Shenzhen, China.

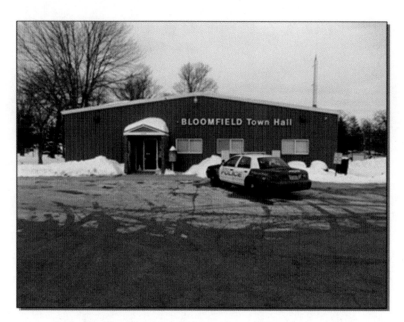

Bloomfield Township Board Supervisor

Southeast, WI

I served ~ 4 years, running for election twice, and winning each time. My productive relations with police, trustees, village president, etc. helped improve local government services.

***

I enjoyed every moment of my life, filled with challenge and achievement. In reflection, I can only say, live the best you can - now. Don't wait for time, people, events to motivate you. You may never capture opportunity on your terms.

Epilogue

After my aneurysm in 2006, not wanting to spend one minute lamenting over my experience, I went back to the gym. "FITNESS PLUS" magazine caught wind of my recovery and wanted to write my story. For those who want to review this magazine article, go to fitplusmag.com.

Their journalist, Tony Padegimas from Fitness Plus, interviewed me about a year after discharge from Banner Good Samaritan Hospital in downtown Phoenix. I've included the article below.

Constant, Steady Steps, March 2007

Her "tip-top" physical condition has made her recovery a lot easier.

***

Background

Francine Merkel still offers her left hand when she meets people. Her right hand isn't up to it, yet. Last winter, she and her husband, Victor, moved from Bloomfield, Wisconsin to Tolleson, AZ just west of Phoenix. They've been married for 37 years, have a grown daughter in Pennsylvania, five grandkids and two great-grandchildren.

***

The Challenge

Last March, a blood vessel burst in the left side of her brain while she was working out at the YMCA. "I was on one of their machines when it happened. I had a brain aneurysm. My husband finally got me to a doctor, because at first, I didn't want to go," she says.

"The morning that they did the operation, the doctor came out and said, 'I don't mean to be so grim, but she could die on the table,'" Victor recalls. "We had only been out here 30 days. The only place I knew was the post office. And I thought, wow - I'm going to have to locate a funeral parlor."

After a seven-hour procedure, Merkel's life was saved, but just about everything else was still questionable. "I couldn't talk. I couldn't move. I couldn't do anything," she says. "It was really horrible."

The Turning Point

Merkel remained in the hospital for three months and continued as an outpatient until September. "After that, I decided I was going to get back to working on my body. And that's what I'm doing," she says.

Merkel exercises five days a week. In Wisconsin, she used to walk three miles a day, work out regularly at the local YMCA, and swim in her backyard pool. Her "tip-top physical condition," Victor says, "gave her a better chance of coming back."

Staying Motivated

"I can see that I'm starting to be able to do things," Merkel says. Her right hand still "doesn't work right" and her right leg is still weak as well, but she says that she's making steady progress. She maintains a high protein diet to gain back some of the 35 pounds she lost in the hospital and looks forward to swimming in her pool this summer.

Goals

Merkel hopes to return to her retirement job as a teacher's aide, but notes, "I found out very quickly - that wasn't going to happen yet. I have to be able to walk and talk and that's not all 100 percent, yet."

2021 Update

Fran passed away from pulmonary collapse on a sunny April day in Tolleson, Arizona.

She survived 15 years after her aneurysm by getting up every day and giving her very best.

Fran maintained the financials for Victor's writing business and their personal finances throughout that period.

She controlled her diet with protein, fruits, and vegetables.

Fran remained active until the end, performing aerobic exercises, weightlifting, and even driving the family car.

She also had many friends and stayed in contact with family daily.

Even though Fran's death has wounded me beyond description, I prefer to think of her life, much the same as a Viking warrior, fighting until her last breath.

A reflection on the last days of her life by husband, Victor Merkel.

Art / Photo Credits

Subject/Art By:

Index

stiff neck, 4

subarachnoid hemorrhage, 9, 36, 41

subarachnoid space, 3, 9

swollen legs, 43, 44

Symbicort, 99, 100

therapy, 32, 95, 96, 102, 103

Tony Padegimas, 113

tracheotomy, 26

Trileptal, 46, 47, 48, 98

unruptured brain aneurysm, 2

value of family, 90

vitamins, 57

weakness and numbness, 3, 4

Wisconsin home, xiii

work out a strategy with incentives, 42, 124

X-ray, 12, 80, 85, 87, 102

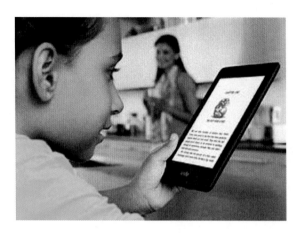

FranGives grants E-READERS to tribal students.

Fran's legacy lives on through FranGives, Inc., 501c3 non-profit. She experienced the blight and neglect of Menominee Tribal Lands and Schools as a child in the 1960s, which fostered a strong empathy later, as a successful Wisconsin lawmaker.

Fran supported legislation to grant food, clothing, and school supplies to schools in need. The FranGives team maintains that same value of empathy to enrich students' lives.

The FranGives program forms partnerships with Arizona tribal and select non-tribal school districts. We foster a commitment in children (ages 4 to 11) that promotes digital skills.

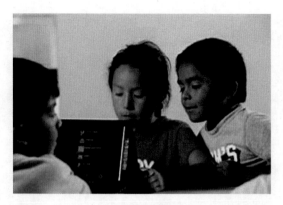

FranGives grants LAPTOPS to tribal students.

FranGives mission is to grow reading proficiency. We grant e-readers, laptops, tablets, iPhones, Chromebooks, and e-books, loaded with incentive-based reading programs.

Today, many tribal elementary and middle school students have not developed digital skills. In those underserved areas, we ensure every student will have access to mobile electronic devices.

Major grants from FranGives to native schools start in fall semesters and continue again in spring semesters. Also, targeted grants are made throughout the school year for conferences, awards, etc.

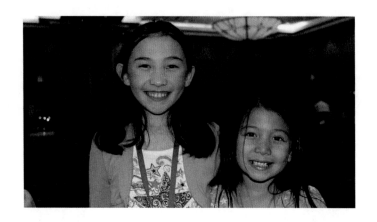

FranGives supports First Nations Development Institute.

Current Initiatives - improve the lives of Navajo, Hopi, San Juan, Pima, and other tribal students.

Perform needs assessments, analyze results, plan/implement fundraising, issue purchase orders to Amazon, Samsung, HP, AZURE distributors.

FranGives looks for low-income areas with limited access to educational resources. We also emphasize schools with low academic performance or high dropout rates.